This book is the future of medicine. It shows how the body works and how physical ailments are the symptom, not the problem. Then it shows specific action steps that will allow the body to heal itself. I recommend this book to anyone interested in a healthy life.

—Bill Ferguson
Author and creator of *Mastery of Life*

As an allopathic medical doctor trained in Physical Medicine and Rehabilitation, I have been trained in working with a team of clinicians to optimize the functional recovery of patients who have become disabled due to injury or illnesses. More recently, I have completed a fellowship in Integrative Medicine, and my eyes have been opened to the benefits of holistic modalities addressing the mind-body-spirit connection. Your Body is a Self-Healing Machine Trilogy *is a perfect guide to those who want to partake in self-care and be co-creators of health and wellness. Especially in the current times, we live where we are constantly challenged to maintain our health, and this information is needed to reverse the damage we have done to our bodies and our environment.*

Understanding why our current health system is not working and why more people are getting sicker as our cost gets exponentially out of control is crucial to becoming empowered to initiate a change. This book gives us an excellent introduction to applied epigenetics and how we can use it to support our self-healing machine that can rebuild itself. Included are practical recommendations on making the optimal nutritional choices, detoxification, lifestyle choices, and addressing the emotional, mental, and spiritual body.

Our bodies need support for healing, but what is often not discussed is what we can do to prevent illness development in the first place. Understanding applied epigenetics will allow each of us to be proactive in our self-care and be part of the solution to our burgeoning healthcare crises. This book will be an excellent resource for my patients and those who want to improve their overall well-being. Before it is too late, we need to spread this valuable information to as many people as possible. Thank you, Dr. Siton, for writing our manual for optimal health!

— Dr. Nelson Valena, MD
Physiatrist
Physician Director of Rehabilitation
Nexus Neurorecovery Center

Gigi Siton, DPT, has truly given us a gift, a plethora of information on how to take care of ourselves. The extensive research behind all the topics that are discussed results in powerful new habits that can completely change our life! I highly recommend everyone to thoroughly read this book to give yourself a new lease on life and to achieve a happier and healthier future.

—Isabelle Valentine
CEO and Entrepreneur
Montessori Schools
Copenhagen, Denmark

Your Body Is a
SELF-HEALING
MACHINE

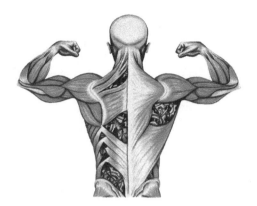

Your Body Is a
SELF-HEALING
M A C H I N E

Understanding Epigenetics
Why It Is Important to Know
BOOK 1

Gigi Siton, DPT
Doctor of Physical Therapy

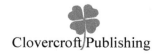

Clovercroft Publishing

Your Body Is a Self-Healing Machine: Understanding Epigenetics, Why Is it Important to Know, Book 1

Published by Clovercroft Publishing, Franklin, Tennessee

Edited by OnFire Books

Copy Edited by Lee Titus Elliott

Cover and Interior Design by Adept Content Solutions

Book Cover Graphics by Patrick Joven

Printed in the United States of America

ISBN: Hardcover 978-1-950892-70-9
        Trade Paperback 978-1-950892-69-3

*This book is lovingly dedicated
to the memory of my amazing parents:*

"Papa George" Attorney George Laurie Siton, Sr.

and

"Mama Liling" Eligia Flores Siton.

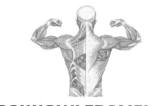

ACKNOWLEDGMENTS

Many people in my life have supported me, have believed in me, have given me hope, and have shared with me information that literally changed my life. The list would be extremely long, and I am limited for space, so thanks to everyone who continues to be part of my life. You know who you are. Thank you. Thank you. Thank you!

I would like to thank my beautiful daughters, Alexandra Siton Till and Victoria Siton Till, for being my inspiration in all that I do.

My thanks to the awesome Holistic Physical Therapy Team, Mylene Thormer BSN, Gary Picar PTA, Andrew Magahis, Tristan Bautista, Mini Puquiz, and Jennifer Osborne; without your unconditional support and commitment day in and day out, there would be no Holistic Physical Therapy Clinic. I thank you for helping people every day recapture their health, for believing and supporting my ideas and vision, and for making this company successful in making the world a healthier place to live!

I thank my dearest sister, Leah Siton Steigerwald, and her husband, Volker Steigerwald, PhD, who tirelessly edited this book while being quarantined in Germany. I thank Doods Siton and Ally Till for helping with book formatting. And, finally, I thank Lisa Capallia and Helen Conol for reviewing my book. I thank

Patrick J. Joven for drawing a masterpiece, the beautiful Self-Healing Body on the book cover.

To all my family and friends too many to mention, thank you for your support in my personal and professional life.

And, of course, I thank Mark Loughead, my biggest support, who got this book out of my head and into my hands.

Maraming Salamat Po!

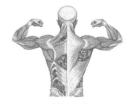

SERIES CONTENTS

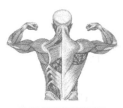

CONTENTS

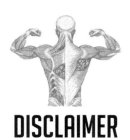

DISCLAIMER

This book is designed to provide helpful information on the subjects discussed. This book is not meant to be used, nor should it be used, to diagnose or to treat any psychological or medical condition. For diagnosis or treatment of any psychological or medical issue, consult your physician. The publisher and the author are not responsible for any specific health needs that may require medical supervision and are not liable for any damages or negative consequences from any treatment, action, application, or preparation to any person reading or following the information in this book. The author and the publisher refuse any and all warranties, liabilities, losses, costs, claims, demands, suits, and actions of any type or nature whatsoever, arising from or in any way related to this book. References are provided for informational purposes only and do not constitute an endorsement of any books, websites, or other sources. Readers should be aware that the websites listed in this book might change. Neither the publisher nor the author shall be liable for any physical, psychological, emotional, financial, or commercial damages, including, but not limited to, special, incidental, consequential, or other damages. The readers are responsible for their own choices, actions, and results.

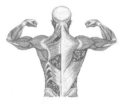

PROLOGUE

I n 1903, Thomas Edison was concerned about the health care of his time and stated: *"The doctor of the future will give no medicine, but will interest his patient in the care of the human frame, in diet and the cause and prevention of disease."* I suspect that he was referring to epigenetics. I truly believe in this statement. For more than thirty years, I have worked as a licensed physical therapist to help people feel better. Epigenetic healing is what drives me passionately about my mission.

Pursuing my mission gave me the chance to help my childhood friend and biggest inspiration for this book, Cyd. We have been best friends since kindergarten in my hometown, Oroquieta City, Philippines. In 2016, she had been working as a financial auditor for almost seventeen years in San Antonio, Texas, but we have kept in touch with each other regularly by phone, and she visits at least twice a year.

In the spring of 2016, she called with urgency in her voice. I knew this was not one of our girlie chitchat calls. She had seen one of my backyard photos I posted while studying epigenetics and nutritional medicine. She proceeded to tell me about her recent diagnoses of kidney, lung, brain, and liver cancers. I immediately requested her medical records. That night, I stayed awake all night long, reading her medical files over and over again. I learned that her cancer was between stages three and four. Her kidney cancer had metastasized in her lungs, in her liver, in her remaining left kidney, and maybe even in her brain. My heart sunk; she must be so scared.

The next day, when we spoke, she asked me if I had reviewed her medical records. With a heavy heart, I asked her if she knew the stage of her cancer. She did not give a clear answer. I had a suspicion that, at this point, she did not want to know every detail of her cancer. I honored her wishes and decided not to tell her what was documented in her medical records. I just let her tell me her story.

She told me that her doctor had removed her right kidney a few months before. She was too weak to qualify for chemotherapy and radiation. She said that her oncologist had sent her home to prepare proper arrangements with her family to be ready for the soon-coming *inevitable day*. The oncologist had said for her to come back in six months, if she was still around. He had given her a dire prognosis of about three to six months to live. With her crackling voice, she sheepishly asked me if I could help her. Every cell of my body wanted to hug her and to make her feel better. I said, *"Of course, I will!"* I was so honored to have been asked to be her healing partner on her cancer journey. I would do my best to help her. So, with tears in our eyes, we decided to move forward right away.

To make matters worse, her husband had also been diagnosed with a very fragile heart condition, almost at the same time. He could not drive or take care of her. So, for the first time, despite being in severe, constant agonizing pain from her cancer, Cyd bravely drove herself the three-hour journey to Houston from San Antonio. She had to make multiple stops to catch her breath because the pain was so unbearable. I was so proud that she did not get lost on the way, and I felt so relieved when her car was pulling up in my driveway. Thank God she arrived safely at my clinic!

Every day, I coached her extensively about applied epigenetics, using nutritional therapy, fasting, and the whole metabolic approach to cancer combined with daily holistic physical therapy and acupuncture to stimulate her immune system. We laughed. We cried.

After one week, she felt so much better and felt confident enough to continue the treatments on her own at home. When we said our good-byes that day, there was a lump in my throat and a deep, dark fear in my heart. Reality hit me like a brick. It dawned on me that this could be the last time I would see her alive. I hugged her so tightly. I suspected she felt the same way because she hugged me back tightly, too. We lingered with our tight hugs. We looked in each other's eyes and nervously giggled, as if we were kids again. I tried to have a brave, happy face for her, but I could not help crying. I could not stop myself from crying. I could feel the huge teardrops running down my cheeks, as I waved good-bye and watched her sweet, smiling face in the car window, as she drove away from the clinic parking lot. We both desperately prayed: "God, help us!"

With a new commitment to life, she vigorously adhered to her holistic treatments at home. Every day, she was feeling better and better. After five months, she had to go to the dreaded oncology workup. We held our breath for the results. After the visit to her oncologist, she was bursting out with joy and excitement. She could not wait to tell me that her doctor could not find any trace of cancer in her lung, in her liver, in her brain, or even in her left kidney. All her organs were functioning 100 percent and were cancer free! Hallelujah! To this day, she continues to apply all the epigenetic principles of healing. I feel honored to be a part of her healing journey. My own childhood best friend is back and well! Thank you, God!

Another holistic physical therapy patient of mine, a seventy-eight-year-old charming and intelligent retired chemical engineer, had been diagnosed with rheumatoid arthritis (RA) for thirteen years. He hobbled into my PT clinic with his very caring wife after his rheumatologist referred him to our clinic. For the previous six years, his wife had needed to help him more and more around the house because of constant, severe joint pains, which were worse in the mornings. He was so unstable and shaky because of severe generalized muscle weakness. The first initial PT evaluation was a little hairy. He almost walked out with his wife after I had talked about our holistic and epigenetic approach to physical therapy. After a good conversation about epigenetics and the biophysics of healing, I was able to appeal to his engineering mind. He began to open up and to embrace the epigenetic and comprehensive approach to healing. After one week of giving up his morning coffee, practicing proper hydration, and drinking his green smoothie daily, he reported that he noticed that his joint pain had been dramatically reduced from eight out of ten on a ten-point scale, to two out of ten. In just two weeks, he could drive on his own and could work on more projects in his workshop. Today, he has no pain anywhere in his body, and he continues to work on core muscle strength and balance. He drives himself to the Holistic PT Clinic. He has even volunteered with his wife in Louisiana for two weeks to help rebuild a church. This is the best, satisfying feeling. I have hundreds, or even thousands, of happy stories like this from our patients. It may take another book to write about all of them.

These experiences are the reason why I wrote this book. I found my passion and my purpose in life: to spread how amazing the concepts of epigenetics are, to take applied epigenetics concepts from the ivory tower of the academics down to a practical and straightforward everyday healthy habit. Epigenetics will last. This is not a fad or a new concept. Epigenetics is as dependable as gravity. It is a given. You must work with it. You cannot ignore this fundamental epigenetic concept that runs in your DNA.

With all modesty, I wrote the trilogy of "Your Body Is A Self-Healing Machine" with you, the non-medical reader, in mind.

Even though these books are packed with ample scientific research and published peer-reviewed medical journals from around the world, I tried to write in a conversational style, infused with many of my personal stories to unravel the beautiful science of epigenetics.

Your body and its self-healing capacity are the true wonders of the world. We heal; however, it is massively dependent on our epigenetic gene expression. The outline of the three books is to highlight the amazingly powerful self-healing capacity of your body. It is divided into three significant parts. Book One is about the introduction of epigenetics and its concepts, holistic healing, and what causes diseases. Book Two is about your body's self-healing systems made up from the primary unit, the cell, and all the multi-immune systems. And finally, Book Three is about what tweaks on or off your gene expression. It is the editing and updating of epigenetic information from environmental factors. This is the applied epigenetics in action. It is your lifestyle choices, which include your nutrition, your hydration, sleeping habits, fresh air, consistent detox, and fasting practice, sun exposure, and your emotional and mental state.

Just as is pictured in my book cover, you are a very efficient self-healing machine. How you run the machine toward health or illness is 100 percent in your control. These three books are my humble attempt to write the basic epigenetic manual for your body. Epigenetic basics are more about your free will and less about your inherent genetic traits. You are not a victim of your genetics. Even if your DNA blueprint is permanent, only you can shape your life. You are the driver of your gene expression. It is massively dependent on your minor or major decisions, either conscious or unconscious. Your daily epigenetic choices will define your health or your disease. What you eat, breathe, or drink; how you sleep; how much you are exposed to sunlight; how you detox and fast— these comprise all the epigenetic information that tweaks your gene expression to turn *on* or *off*. You are what you eat, breathe, feel, and think! Applied epigenetics are the little things that make a significant impact on your overall health. I hope and pray that, after reading this book, you can start implementing them one at a time, until you can create your own healthy habits.

If you want to improve your health and understand epigenetics healing, this book is for you. This trilogy book is based on my Epigenetics 101 class. I have students as young as ten years old and as old as eighty-nine years old. Elementary school students, school principals, businesspeople, CEOs, homemakers, teachers, nurses, physical therapists, and medical doctors have attended the class. Wives drag their husbands to participate in the study, and, in the end, the husbands were glad they came. I invite you to attend as a couple or as a group because I believe in a team approach to healing. It's good to have a healing buddy on your journey.

My mission is to make epigenetics become a movement, beyond cultural and geographical boundaries. More important, it will become a significant factor in the practice of medicine. I wish to inspire you to become passionate and to practice applied epigenetics in your daily life. I hope and pray to make a massive life-changing impact one reader at a time. This is my way to make epigenetics spread like wildfire, and I invite you to go along on this journey with me!

A BRIEF STORY ABOUT MY BACKGROUND

Growing up, my family lived in the provincial town and grew our garden; every meal was home-cooked, and we did not even have electricity. Back then, we were called poor, and now we are called organic! We had no refrigerator, so everything we ate was fresh. Even though we did not grow up wealthy, we made do with what we had. We built our home on the weekends for almost five years—the whole family, kids, and all, making enough concrete bricks for our house.

My parents and my eleven siblings modeled a life of service, academic excellence, strong faith, and love. Both of my parents had humble beginnings. My father worked as a janitor to pay for his college and a pre-law degree. He worked his way up so that he became the dean of the college of law in the same school. He was also a full-time criminal lawyer and state prosecutor in our local province. My father's family comes from a long line of ancient healers and herbalists from Siquijor Island. My mother was a coconut-processing factory worker during her teens in our hometown. She finished a graduate degree in special education and worked as a supervisor in elementary education. My parents were healthy, and both had healthy mind-sets.

My most beautiful memory of my parents was when they were ballroom dancing on the dance floor. They enjoyed dancing with each other. My father had nine daughters, so after he danced with my mother, he would pick one of us girls to dance next. Dancing with him was such a treat that he made you feel amazing; he would say, "Oh, you're a good dancer!" He was a true renaissance man; he was a self-taught intellectual. He was always smiling, and he laughed a lot. He could hang out with fishermen, as well as with the prominent dignitaries. He treated them all the same, very kind and humble. My father swam two miles in the ocean almost every day, worked in his garden, and maintained our private beachfront with his bare hands, not to mention that he had two full-time jobs!

My mother was a local beauty queen in our home town. She fell in love with my father at the very young age of eighteen. She had eleven home-birthed children, all of whom became well-educated. She had a formidable spirit. I will always remember her jovial presence with contagious laughter whenever she is around. She went back to finish college and went on to earn her graduate degree in education after her eighth child. With my father's meager income, she was the best economist and financial manager for the

Siton tribe. She had a quiet grace and a powerful strength next to my father. She was able to juggle her career and managed to take care of her twelve children, including at least ten to twenty extended family at a time, who were living with us.

When I was twenty years old and in my senior year in pre-med school (psychology at University of Santo Tomas, in Manila), my life changed dramatically. One fateful night in August 1985, on his way home while on his bike after teaching night class, my father was brutally assassinated for his noble work in fighting corruption. He had been a state prosecutor in the Provincial Fiscal Office in Oroquieta City, Philippines. In his seven-day wake, the entire town mourned. The heartfelt tribute came from every corner of the country; rich and poor came; on foot, on tricycles, on buses, in canoes, in cars, and by planes. He was honored and well-loved by everyone. His funeral procession went on for miles and took the whole day because everyone wanted to pay their respect to my father.

Sadly, after two years, my mother joined my father in heaven. She died in her sleep of a broken heart after my father died. Because both of my parents were gone, I had to say good-bye to my dream of becoming a doctor. I had to regroup and considered another career option in the medical field. I did the next best thing and went to physical therapy school in De La Salle-EAC Dasmarinas, Cavite. After three years, I was directly hired and headed to the United States as a physical therapist in Conroe, Texas, in 1989. The rest is history.

Interestingly, my life has come full circle, preparing me for my career in teaching epigenetics. I started my college education in engineering, so I had a solid foundation in sciences and physics. Then, I wanted to be a medical doctor, so I took a bachelor of science in psychology as a pre-med. My psychology training helped me appreciate the power of a person's belief system and how it massively affects the physical body. Then, fate intervened.

I lost my parents, so being a medical doctor was not an option for me any longer. I had to make a little detour and went to physical therapy. Being trained in physical therapy gave me a good grasp of human anatomy and the biophysics of movement. It gave me the tools on how to help patients recover and restore function. Initially, I thought my engineering and psychology background would be useless; however, all three disciplines played a significant role in the whole integrated healing approach. I never realized that my humble beginnings and my entire educational journey prepared me for an epic journey in epigenetics. Amazingly, the universe had planned my life path long before I knew the significance of it. This is truly a classic example that there is no accident in life. My whole career is genuinely serendipitous!

Your Body Is a

SELF-HEALING

M A C H I N E

TRILOGY

Understanding Epigenetics
Why It Is Important to Know
BOOK 1

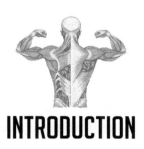

INTRODUCTION

W hat if I told you that everything you were taught about genetics for the past 100 years is faulty. Suppose I told you that everything you knew about your diet, health, and disease were also wrong. We have all been misled unintentionally and intentionally. For decades, I, like everyone else, believed all the lies. I was taught that whatever my parents had, I was destined to get as well. Whether I liked it or not, I was a victim of my inherited genes. Therefore, my best chance for survival was in the medical doctors' capable hands; that is it. Doctors knew best. So, I joined the medical profession as a physical therapist with a burning desire to heal. I believed everything I learned in physical therapy school was the best that science could offer. But the moment I started working with my patients, there was a nagging voice inside my head that kept asking the same question, "If I am doing everything I know to be right, why was I just managing pain symptoms and not addressing the cause of the problem?"

Perhaps you have suffered for some time a nagging pain in your neck, low back, headaches, aching joints, morning stiffness, hyperacidity, or a myriad of digestive conditions that you cannot shake. Perhaps you have been diagnosed with a chronic degenerative illness that your doctor convinced you is a part of the aging process, like osteoarthritis or bulging disc disease. Maybe you also suffer from one or more autoimmune diseases, type 1 or type 2 diabetes, metabolic syndrome, thyroid or hormonal imbalances, asthma, allergies, or even cancer. You probably know that something is not right, but you do not know what. Maybe you have tried all those medications conventional medicine can offer, but you are still suffering. Worse, perhaps the treatments are making you sicker with new symptoms. You probably surrendered that you are doomed to take all the pills your doctor prescribed for the rest of your life. Adding guilt to your heavy load, you blame your parents' genes and surrender to the fact you are a victim of your genetic inheritance. So, why try to eat healthy when you are doomed with the same outcome. Sadly, you are not alone in this mess.

Does this sound awfully familiar?

Being a victim and hearing this victimhood dilemma from my patients did not sit well with me. So, I started researching the best way to achieve optimal health. About twenty years ago, I encountered the concept of epigenetics. With my engineering, psychology, and thirty-two years of clinical experience in physical therapy, epigenetics provided solid scientific clarity to what were very complex health issues and diseases. It all made so much sense to me!

If you, too, feel like a victim of your genes, all that is about to change for you. Epigenetics to the rescue! Let us start by saying, "My body is a self-healing machine!" Let us stop blaming our parents' genes and start making good healthy choices to support our health and our immune system's destiny. That is right; you are in control of your health as well as your illness. Your doctor is just your assistant to your health journey. Repeat after me: "I am made perfect. Inside of me is a self-healing machine!"

I have the solution for you in this trilogy. But first, you must let go of everything you have learned about your body, your health, and your diet from conventional Western medicine. You must be ready to undo all your old assumptions about what you were taught about healthy life and healing. I read somewhere that unlearning is the highest form of learning. I am aware that it is twice as hard to correct outdated concepts as learning new ones. This first book in the trilogy is packed with practical and logical health information that will dispel myths ingrained in our traditional Western medical sciences. It will challenge your core beliefs on health and healing deeply. I will introduce basic biophysics concepts that may initially blow your mind and turn everything you thought you knew upside down. But here is the excellent news: knowing epigenetics concepts will empower you. I will reveal how amazing your body is, what makes it work, and how to keep it healthy. Once you remove your outdated health myths and academic roadblocks, nothing is standing in the way of vibrant health. The fear of the dreaded inherited illnesses will be conquered, and your life will change for the better.

I wrote book one to unravel epigenetics' basic concepts. It will show clarity on why it is essential to apply epigenetics in our daily lives. This book also provides a greater understanding of your bio-individual metabolic physiology. I utilized the simple analogy for your body as a self-healing machine. This way, it is easier to unlock its basic concepts and epigenetics principles into more usable and compelling self-healing tools for your health. Epigenetics is more about your personal choices and less about your inherent genetic traits. You are not a victim of your genetics. Instead, you are the driver of your gene expression. Your choices can turn your gene expression *off* or *on*! It is massively dependent on the consequences of your minor and major decisions, either consciously or unconsciously. Your daily epigenetic choices define your health or disease.

More importantly, understanding gene expression only highlights the tragic dilemma of modern medicine. "Death by

Medicine" is a sad reality, one in which we have become far too complacent. Besides, we have to face the devastating consequence of the twenty-first century worldwide epidemic of poly-pharmacy syndromes. There is an urgent need for epigenetics in our current health care system. This book will offer a simple solution found in its foundational healing principles. It also explains the rationale for why we need to honor pain as a loyal messenger, not the enemy of the body. We must learn to listen to our body's early warning system, like pain, and respond with epigenetics concepts and practical principles.

You will essentially learn that the major causes of degenerative diseases can be categorized as either: (1) congestion/stagnation, and (2) depletion/deficiency. Understanding the causes of illness from a biophysics perspective will clearly show that optimal health maintenance, and prevention is so natural and attainable. In most illnesses, there are the primary or mother conditions where most degenerative diseases originate. If left unresolved, secondary symptoms will develop as a result of prolonged primary disorders. Being aware of the initial or mother conditions and acting on the early stages will address the problem's root. It will give your body the best advantage to reverse disease and restore health. The epigenetics way empowers you to know your body and to act responsibly.

Finally, this book addresses the appalling effects of environmental and human-made toxins. The pervasive and subtle exposure of toxins in every aspect of our daily lives could cause massive harm to your health by turning your gene expression for illness. Sadly, these permanent adverse effects on the gene expression can be transmitted to the next multi-generations to come.

Let us put epigenetics at the forefront of the twenty-first century. This book *"Understanding Epigenetics—Why It Is Important To Know"* from the trilogy *"Your Body Is A Self-Healing Machine"* will provide the roadmap to optimal health prevention and maintenance, and maybe even to cure!

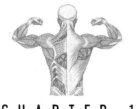

CHAPTER 1

WHAT IS EPIGENETICS?

"The natural healing force within each one of us is the greatest force in getting well."
—Hippocrates

E *pigenetics* is the most compellingly practical and effective healing paradigm to date. The prefix *epi* comes from the Greek word meaning *on top of or in addition to*. *Genetics* is derived from the Greek word *genetikos*, meaning *origin*, and *Genetics* is now known as the scientific study of heredity. Heredity refers to the genetic properties or characteristics of an organism, including human beings.

In this book, I am referring to the epigenetics of healing and illness. Epigenetics is the influence of your environment that greatly affects your genetic expression either for health or illness. It is not about your physical or your hereditary attributes. It refers to the external factors that tweak your DNA to turn genes *on* or *off*. These external factors cannot rearrange the DNA sequence; instead, they affect how cells *read* genes.[1]

Imagine that you have an identical twin, your genetic clone. However, you were each raised in a separate environment. What if one of you was raised in a good, nurturing neighborhood while your twin sibling was raised in a bad, toxic neighborhood? What do you think would happen after fifty years? You and your twin would probably look very different from each another in your health, your mind-set, and your overall outlook on life. It turns out that you and your twin would also be totally different individuals inside. If both of your genetic codes were tested, the result of your DNA would still be the same as your twin's. For example, pretend that your genome is a paragraph; you and your twin have all the words in the same sequence of letters. Yet, there is a huge difference. You could say that the letters are in the same order but that the spaces and the punctuation are all in different places. Of course, it will entirely change the message of that paragraph.

The study of this epigenetic punctuation is called "epigenetics." It means "above your genomes." The epigenome does not mess with your DNA blueprint, but it does decide or control the degree to which or whether some genes are expressed in different cells in

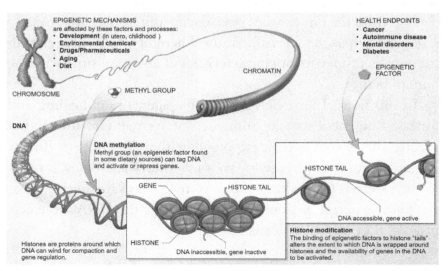

FIGURE 1. Epigenetics

your body. The study of epigenetics looks at changes to your genes throughout your entire life and whether those changes could be passed on to your children or even your grandchildren.

So here is how epigenetics works. Your body has trillions of cells. They each contain your DNA, the same blueprint of your genetic code. Your physical traits, like your genetic race, your hair color, and the height that you were born with, are pretty much a given, and you cannot change them. You can change and improve your body's DNA gene expression, either in health or in illness. Your DNA does not automatically know what to do with your body. Your DNA needs outside instructions from these little carbon and hydrogen compounds called "methyl groups." Methyl groups control the genome by tagging to a gene and by saying, "Do not express this gene." These methyl groups bind differently to your genome. Your DNA tells your immature cells what their job is going to be in the body, like, *"Hey, you are going to be a bone cell!"* or, *"Hey, you are going to a muscle cell."*

In addition to the methyl groups, *histones* also control your epigenetics. Histones are proteins that are the spools of DNA that wind themselves around. Histones can change how tightly or how loosely your DNA is wound around them. If they are more loosely wound, then your genes can express more, and if they are more tightly wound, then your genes can express less. Think of the methyl group like a switch and the histones like a turning knob. Every cell of your body has a distinct methylation-and-histone pattern. That is what gives every cell its marching orders.

Consider your DNA genomes as the actual hardware of your computer. Your epigenome is more like the software that tells the hardware what to do. So, your genome will be doing all the cell work, but it needs your epigenome to tell your DNA what to do. As the hardware, your DNA will be the same throughout your life, but your epigenetic tags can change throughout your life. The epigenetic tags decide what genes get expressed or what genes do not get expressed. The good thing is that this epigenetic information in a cell is not permanent. It changes throughout your life; a change that is 100 percent within your control.

Your epigenetic tags can be inherited, or they can change over time, especially when your body is going through a lot of changes. During puberty, your methyl groups will kick into high gear, affecting your hormonal changes. Or, when you get pregnant, your epigenome must be fully engaged to develop a baby. This is where the mother's epigenetic environment is very critical. Your baby is brewing in your maternal swimming pool, called *amniotic fluid*. The quality of the maternal fluid is a product of the mother's diet, hydration, sleep, stress, and all the environmental factors surrounding the pregnancy. You could say that these environmental factors will influence the punctuation of the baby's genetic codes that are passed down before the baby is born. Nevertheless, not only in these exciting times are the epigenomes formed; but they also continuously get edited or updated throughout our entire lives. These changes vary, based on environmental factors, like what we do, what we eat, what we smoke, and how stressed we are every day. I daresay that your health or diseases are passed down mainly by recipes, not entirely by genes. If you eat like your parents, the more likely you will get the same conditions they experience.

Studies have found that environmental factors, like bad diets, can lead the methyl groups to bind in the wrong places and to make mistakes by giving bad instructions to your genes. These cells with bad instructions become abnormal, and malfunction occurs. When that happens, all the cellular messages go haywire and become diseased or, even worse, cancerous.

A BRIEF HISTORY OF EPIGENETICS

Generations of scientists and the public have been taught genetics, but few have been exposed to the relatively new science of epigenetics – in fact, the inclusion of epigenetics into the molecular elements of biology and evolution has been met with opposition.[2] Epigenetics is a relatively very young science, even though we have known about the epigenome since the 1930s.

Fifty years before Charles Darwin, Jean-Baptiste Lamarck proposed *"that the environment can directly alter traits, which are then inherited by generations to come."* [3] Lamarck, a professor of invertebrate zoology at the National Museum of Natural History in Paris, studied many organisms including insects and worms in the late eighteenth and early nineteenth centuries.[4] He introduced the words "biology" and "invertebrate" into the scientific lexicon, and wrote books on biology, invertebrates, and evolution.[2] Sadly, despite his significant academic career, for 200 years Lamarck's theory had been long relegated in the back shelves of academic scientific studies.

In the 1950s, James Watson and Francis Crick were able to explain the mysteries of DNA and the double helix. In that same year, the developmental biologist Conrad Waddington of the University of Edinburgh, coined a modern term—*epigenetics*— to describe this phenomenon of rapid change. He reported that fruit flies exposed to an outside chemical stimulus or changes in temperature during embryonic development could be pushed to develop varying wing structures. He observed that environmental factors could directly impact physical traits. The changes the scientists induced in that single generation would, thereafter, be inherited to multiple unexposed generations.[2]

Methylation and other epigenetic reactions influence health and disease processes across generations. In the 2000s, Michael Skinner, PhD, and his team at the Washington State University identified pervasive evidence on a non-genetic form of inheritance, called *"epigenetic transgenerational inheritance."* In 2005, his team published their findings in the journal *Science*. The scientific article showed the ability of environmental chemicals to promote the inheritance of disease in rats through three generations, to great-grand offspring and beyond, in the absence of any continued exposures.[5] Ancestral exposure to environmental influences, such as toxicants, abnormal nutrition, or stress, can induce changes in the germline epigenome that are transmitted to descendants. Ultimately, epigenetic transgenerational inheritance (ETI) will increase disease susceptibility of future generations of offsprings.[5]

The phenomenon has been further documented by many labs in a number of different species over the past decade. An example is when Graham Burdge and his team at the University of Southampton in the United Kingdom reported that excessive nutrition in rats created epigenetically induced metabolic abnormalities three generations out.[6] In 2011, a study by Sibum Sung and his colleagues at the University of Texas, Austin, found that drought and changes in temperature induced epigenetic evolution in plants, leading to alterations in growth and flowering traits, generations out.[7] Another study, conducted in 2012 by Gerlinde Metz and her colleagues at the University of Lethbridge in Canada found strong evidence on the impact of transgenerational programming versus life-long experience on health and disease. This study demonstrated that restraining pregnant rats or, alternatively, forcing them to swim, produced epigenetic damage that put newborns at risk. This ancestral stress also promoted the ETI of abnormalities in the great-grand offspring of the exposed gestating female.[8]

Environmentally induced epigenetic transgenerational inheritance has now been observed in plants, insects, fish, birds, rodents, pigs,[9] and humans.[10] The ETI of phenotypic trait variation and disease has been shown to occur across a span of at least ten generations in most organisms, with the most extensive studies done in plants for hundreds of generations.[2]

Lamarck was right on the fact that environmental factors can directly alter our biology, even in the absence of direct and continued exposure. Sadly, the altered biology, as seen on the altered genetic expression of traits or in the form of disease can be transmitted from one generation and beyond. If the effects of exposure can indeed be transmitted to subsequent generations, this would have major public health implications; therefore, it is critical to determine how widespread and robust the phenomenon.

It is important to highlight the book written in the 1930s, *Pottenger's Cats: A Study in Nutrition* by Francis Marion Pottenger, Jr., MD. Dr. Pottenger's study was a ten-year comparative study of healthy cats between those fed with raw foods and those fed with cooked foods. He studied both cats fed with raw food and cats fed with cooked foods: their behavioral characteristics, their arthritis, their sterility, their skeletal deformities, and their allergies, which are some of the conditions associated with consuming cooked foods. He extensively studied four generations of 900 cats, and he noted the differences in metabolic effects between the cats fed with raw food and the cats fed with cooked food. The cats fed with meals consisting of one-third unpasteurized milk, two-thirds uncooked meat, and cod liver oil were healthy during their entire life spans. Incidentally, healthy plants thrived in the cat pens filled with uncooked food; in contrast, nothing grew in the cat pens filled with cooked food. The cats who ate cooked food, pasteurized milk, evaporated milk, and sweetened condensed milk were smaller and sicker. These cats showed multiple deformities and deficiencies in their faces, their muscles, their skeletons, their fur, and their brains, compared to the cats fed with uncooked food.

All three generations of cats fed with uncooked food were healthy, while the first generation of cats fed with cooked food became sick with degenerative diseases in late life. The second generation of cats fed with cooked food became sick with degenerative diseases in midlife. The third generation of cats fed with cooked food became sick with degenerative diseases in infancy with conditions such as spontaneous abortion, infertility, cancer, arthritis, juvenile diabetes, and hypertension. The good news is that all degenerative diseases were reversed when the fourth generation of cats fed with cooked food was reintroduced to a proper cat diet, consisting of uncooked or raw food. After seventy-four years, this long-term comparative study is still very relevant in epigenetics today.

Only within the last twenty years have we even known what effect these epigenetics tags are having on our DNA. Until that time, scientists still thought that our epigenetics tags were stripped off our genome before they were passed to our children. So, if you started eating lousy food when you were ten years old or if you started taking birth control pills at eighteen, those would certainly be a horrible health decision for you. You would not necessarily be harming your unborn children right away; however, this way of thinking is changing pretty rapidly. Recent epigenetics studies have validated that most of the epigenetics information from a parent is stripped off from the embryo's genome in the first few days and new ones are created for this new person. Yet studies have also shown that some of these tags can be stuck on the genome and passed down from generation to generation. This is a whole new way of thinking about how we give information between ages. Your grandmother did not realize that she was making dietary decisions that could affect you today. Just as in Dr. Pottenger's cat study from one generation to another, epidemics of diabetes, autoimmune disorders, and cancers were not appearing in previous generations. Now you can see type 2 diabetes in younger and younger children. It is starting to look like these illnesses were caused by epigenetics information passed down from the parents.

In the 1980s, it was discovered that environmental factors and your parents' experiences could be passed down from generation to generation. Some scientists were looking at the birth and death records of people who lived in Norrbotten, Sweden, in the nineteenth century. Norrbotten is the northernmost county in Sweden, literally in the Arctic Circle. Its residents were very isolated from the rest of the world, living only by farming. They sustained themselves entirely on the plants they grew and on the farm animals they raised. If they didn't have a good harvest, they died of starvation. Sometimes, when they had a bountiful harvest, food was everywhere. The Swedish public health specialists and scientists looked at the effects on the people who grew up during the periods of bad harvests versus those who grew up during the periods of good harvests. The scientists found that the people of Norrbotten lived their lives in a relentless seasonal cycle of having relatively less to eat to having relatively more to eat than they needed. On average, the people who over-ate died six years sooner than their starved counterparts.

Epigenetics brings both bad news and good news. The bad news is that most of these degenerative diseases are mainly your fault. In addition, scientists found that misplaced epigenetic tags could cause certain types of cancer. Environmental factors, like a lousy diet or a poor lifestyle, could misplace these epigenetic tags. A study identified several lifestyle factors that may modify epigenetics patterns: factors such as diet, obesity, physical activity, tobacco smoking, alcohol consumption, environmental pollutants, psychological stress, and working on night shifts.[11] The good news is that new drugs are being developed that can silence the bad genes that were supposed to be turned off in the first place. And the best news of all is that you can turn off degenerative diseases by making healthy and positive epigenetics modifications in your diet, in your lifestyle, and in your mental and spiritual life.

Until the recent discovery of epigenetics, the scientific community told us that genes were all you were destined to be. Your DNA blueprint was permanent, and you could not escape it. The scientific community also suggested a skewed social prejudice when you look at data without considering social and epigenetics factors. For instance, the debate about intelligence genes might indicate that people with less money are less intelligent. Even as recently as fifteen years ago, some scientists were asserting that some people already have good genes for intelligence while poor people did not have good genes for intelligence at all. Thankfully, we now know that this assertion was so wrong. Not only is there a wide variety of social factors that affect how well you do in intelligence tests, how well you do on such tests is also a product of both your genes and your environment. Your genome's fate is determined by any number of decisions made by any number of your ancestors. And the best news? You can still make positive decisions that are going to affect your health right now, as well as the health of generations beyond your lifetime.

APPLIED EPIGENETICS

Applied epigenetics is the art of moving epigenetics regulation or modification into a more pragmatic and positive approach, to control your gene expression. It is the art of resetting or updating your gene expression by choosing the best epigenetics information from the environment or from your conscious and unconscious response to the environment. Applied epigenetics, correctly practiced, is potentially the most significant breakthrough in the fields of health and longevity to date. This approach empowers us to know how our environment affects us and how to make positive choices that activate our genetic potential for our health and our well-being.

The quality of the bioelectrical and biochemical signals from the food we eat, from the air we breathe, from the words we speak, and from the environment in which we live influences our epigenetics information, which massively affects our gene expression. Epigenetics turns on and off the DNA expression, either for health or for illness. Additionally, our perceptions of and responses to the world we live in, such as our thoughts, our beliefs, our intentions, our relationships, our emotions, and our prayers influence our internal environment. These factors cause chemical changes in our brains and our bodies. All this epigenetics information affects the way our genes communicate with and instruct our cells. It has the effect of altering and of activating our gene expression.

I agree with Bruce Lipton, PhD, in his book *Biology of Belief.* He delicately contended that your perceptions and your beliefs rule your biology. Your immune system is controlled consciously and unconsciously by your understanding and perceptions of events. Fundamentally, the strength of your positive or negative coping mechanisms impact your immune system.

According to Deepak Chopra, MD, a physician and best-selling author, we can modify our genes and initiate DNA activation through our actions and behaviors. It is what applied epigenetics is all about. After knowing epigenetics, we need to master and to consistently practice its principles to achieve optimal health.

In short, applied epigenetics is the art of practicing epigenetics principles. It is to create a positive impact on our genetic mechanisms, to silence or to express our genes. It should be the first line of preventing disease, of maintaining health, of healing illness. It is proactive health care that educates you about and that empowers you with the art of knowing the basics of the causes of diseases, your body's self-healing system, and your body's self-healing tools. It is essential to emphasize that complete healing does

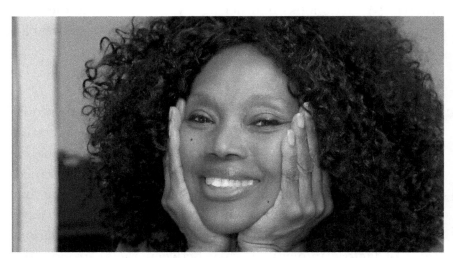

FIGURE 2. The Ageless Lady: Annette Larkins

not happen by accident. It happens through epigenetics! Consistent epigenetic practice is the best way to be healthy and ageless.

A classic example of a person with ageless health and beauty is Annette Larkins. She is an amazing, beautiful seventy-eight-year old lady. She looks and functions like a thirty-year old. She was able to achieve this through a drastic change of diet from the standard American diet to a raw vegan diet at the age of fifty. She was able to slow her aging and to maintain a youthful appearance dramatically. She wears a size four and looks fantastic for her age.

On the other hand, her eighty-four-year-old husband of fifty-two years looks sick and overweight. He takes prescription medicines for his diabetes and high blood pressure. He used to own a meat store and did not change his diet when his wife changed hers. When they are next to each other, they look four decades apart. He said that other people mistake his wife for his granddaughter or that people would ask him the name of the young girlfriend who was with him. It is a classic case of the aging rate difference affected by several epigenetics choices. Both individuals lived under the same roof but chose different lifestyles and nutritional intakes for over fifty years of marriage. The results are massively different. Annette looks half her age with her healthy diet and lifestyle, while her husband has aged so much faster by eating bad foods and by taking medications.

METABOLIC BIO-INDIVIDUALITY

Metabolic bio-individuality means that all humans have their own unique genetic metabolic physiology. A study of your ancestral background can show how you inherently process or metabolize your food—for example, in the classic case of lactose intolerance. Lactose intolerance is a real and crucial clinical syndrome, but its exact prevalence is not known. One estimate puts the average lactose intolerance rate at 65 percent of the global population. Rates of lactose intolerance vary between racial groups; the condition is most common in Africans, Latinos, Asians, and least common in Europeans.[12] Lactose intolerance is caused by a missing enzyme in the gut, called *lactase*. Without that enzyme, lactose in dairy products cannot be metabolized, thereby causing an upset stomach, indigestion, and lots of gassy byproduct.

I have lactose intolerance and a low animal-meat threshold. My genetic metabolic physiology did not change, even though I crossed the Pacific Ocean to immigrate to Texas almost thirty years ago. My lactose intolerance remains. I still suffer from stomach bloating and gassy symptoms every time I drink or eat dairy products.

As for my animal meat consumption, I was used to fresh, wild-caught fish daily. My Filipino metabolic bio-individuality is not geared to overeating meat. I grew up eating simple meals with fresh vegetables, hot soups, and freshly caught fish. My regular diet while I was growing up was all home-cooked and consisted of fresh fish, rice, fresh fruit, and vegetables three times a day, day in and day out. During lean times, fresh vegetables with dried salted fish with lots of rice were the norm. Snacking was not an option. We ate only during family meals, using small plates.

In most authentic rural Filipino dishes, the meat was used only for flavoring. Occasionally, we would feast on pasture-raised chicken or homegrown pork or grass-fed beef, which came from animals raised in our backyard. On special occasions, like town fiestas, Christmases, or birthdays, plenty of meat dishes were served. We would have *Lechon*, a slow open-roasted whole pig, as the centerpiece. Constant meat consumption was too expensive for my parents to be able to feed almost thirty people at a time. Besides my poor economic background, my genetic metabolic bio-individuality may be the reason why too much animal-based meat is hard on my small liver and small stomach. My genetic metabolic physiology is not designed for meat.

There is substantial evidence that people from Asian countries acquire the same disease risk as North Americans when they migrate, mainly because of epigenetics such as diet and lifestyle. According to a 2017 article by Christina Mattina, an editor at *The American Journal of Managed Care*, Filipino Americans over fifty are at a high risk of diabetes, even if they are not obese. This study finds that the prevalence of diabetes is significantly higher among non-obese Filipino Americans aged fifty and older than in their white counterparts, even after controlling for lifestyle factors.[13]

When Filipinos immigrated to the United States, they changed their diet drastically. Besides eating more American food, they still cooked and ate Filipino food, but the ratio between meat and vegetables was not the same. They began eating a massive amount of animal meat in their diet, by three to tenfold, most likely the same serving size and frequency as their American counterparts. Anatomically, Filipinos, male and female, are generally smaller in stature, compared to an average American. Therefore, it is safe to assume that my digestive organs, like my liver, my pancreas, and my stomach, have, on average, a smaller size, compared to the average American. This small-scale digestive system, when consistently overloaded and overworked with the massive standard American serving sizes, will eventually break down and lead to chronic degenerative diseases, like type 2 diabetes. Hence, Filipinos do not have to gain weight to get diabetes. I think the serving sizes for Filipinos should be made according to their ideal body size and bio-individuality.

OLD GENETIC CODE—CONVENTIONAL GENETICS

A fantastic study published in 2017 by Bruce Lipton PhD, described his cloning stem cell research while teaching in a medical school.[14] At that time, the prevailing belief was that genes can turn themselves on and off. The genes regulated not just our physical structure but also our emotions and our behaviors. He wanted to find out what controls our genes. He cloned 50,000 stem cells in a petri dish from the same parent. Then he created three slightly different environments of culture medium in three different petri dishes, with genetically identical cells in each of them. All three developed distinctly, according to the environment they were in, despite the cells having identical genes. As a result, petri dish A turned into muscle cells, petri dish B turned into bone cells, while petri dish C turned into fat cells. He concluded that it is the environment that selects the genetic activity of the cell. It was a total departure from the genetic determinism that he was teaching at that time.

For the past sixty years, the conventional genetic paradigm has taught us that we are victims of our genes. Our physical attributes and diseases are beyond our control; our DNA is powerless against illness. Our free will has a limited impact on our health and immune system. Yes, it is a fact that your physical characteristics are predetermined. You inherit those physical qualities from both parents, including hair color, the color of your skin, height, even personalities, and taste buds. However, your immune capabilities for health and diseases, whether acute or chronic, are not predestined, unless you are born with them. I do not believe that God designed disease pathology to be a cruel legacy of our genetics. I disagree with genetic victimhood.

Just because one of your parents or family members has cancer or a chronic illness does not mean that you will be doomed to have it, as well. This is a myth, and, unfortunately, many people believe it. The truth is that you have the power to determine your health. You can massively change your gene expression when you change your epigenetics mechanisms, like your diet or your lifestyle.

Conventional genetic treatments are performed mainly by using chemicals, drugs, and surgery for most diseases, especially cancer. Recently, the cancer genetic mapping science and technology have advanced exponentially in their specific genetic phenotype profile. Most genetic cancer therapy is based on its genetic cancer profiling. Yet, it does not reveal a complete picture of why and how the patients got cancer. It is like blaming the patient's genetic DNA as the cause of their condition. Cancer's genetic marker is only a symptom of a disease, like the scene of the crime in a criminal investigation. The crime scene, or the genetic cancer profile, is just a clue on what DNA was damaged. It does not necessarily reveal the actual cause. Your genetic profile, either cancer or any neurodegenerative diseases, only reveals your genetic potential. Many factors can cause to activate your cancer potential into a full blown disease. Blaming your genetic profile is like blaming the scene of the crime as the cause of the crime. Your epigenetics mechanisms can silence or activate your inherited genes. Your physical attributes inherited from your parents do not automatically mean that your DNA's expression will behave the same way as that of your parents. One is predetermined, while the latter is very dependent on the epigenetics information that you expose your DNA to throughout your entire life.

Your DNA is permanent, but you can always update or edit your gene expression by making the right choices in your environment every day. Today I try to make the same positive and healthy choices that my parents made, such as dancing. My DNA is strong, but I still do not leave anything to chance. You can't control your blueprint, your DNA, but you can change your gene expression through epigenetics. God gave you your immune system, your age, your hair, your eye color, and your ethnicity. You can't modify them permanently, but you can modify the way you live.

How can you make healthier choices?

Think about the epigenetics implication of cancer or of any diseases, just as the bad choices you made throughout your life can turn on your cancer. You can willfully and continuously turn it off by making smart and intelligent epigenetics choices to silence your cancer or any disease gene expression. You may need help from your doctors to mitigate immediate medical symptoms, but your epigenetics input is the most significant factor in preventing them, and even reversing them.

The problem with the current practice of medicine is the refusal to address the role of epigenetics in the metabolic, lifestyle, and environmental factors that affect health or disease. Knowing the actual cause of a disease will reveal the most useful treatments, especially in degenerative diseases. We need to focus on finding out what triggered the disease gene to express itself and to behave pathologically. Only then can we design an effective intervention strategy or even prevention. Billions of dollars have been spent on the failed symptoms-centered treatments, like cancer studies. This money has not made a dent in the incidence of cancer, even after sixty years of research and development. Since both epigenetics mechanisms and lifestyles are modifiable, they can empower you to be in control and to be the driver of your own DNA expression into illness or, better yet, into health.

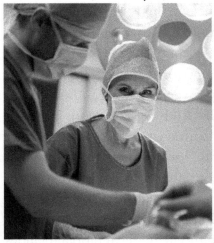

FIGURE 3. Surgery

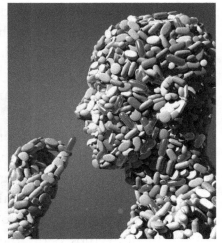

FIGURE 4. Drug Overdose

MODERN MEDICINE'S DILEMMA

Drug overdose deaths continue to impact communities in the United States. According to the Center for Disease Control and Prevention (CDC) data, in its understanding of the epidemic from 1999 to 2017, more than 702,000 people died from an overdose involving any opioid, including prescription and illicit opioids. On average, 130 Americans die every day from an opioid overdose.[15] There is more death because of overdose and overuse of prescription medication than any disease or epidemic.

Sadly, 92.4 percent of U.S. surgeries are deemed unnecessary, and 20 percent are deemed unsuccessful.[16] Unnecessary invasive procedures risk harming patients physically, emotionally, and financially. According to a 2017 study, the researchers systematically searched the literature to identify cases of unnecessary procedures reported from 2008 to 2016.[16] The study found that 92.4 percent of surgeries were performed mainly for financial gain. Surgeons were implementing unnecessary procedures that generated significant revenue well beyond that of standard medical practice. For example, the literature highlighted that the surgeons billed more than $1 million for unnecessary spinal-fusion surgeries.[16] Another major factor was the failure of or the deficient environment for medical oversight mechanisms.[16] There have to be thorough and efficient medical oversight check-and-balance controls to protect patients.

Another study asked the question: "Why do surgeons continue to perform unnecessary surgery?" Researchers found two overarching answers from the study: (1) surgeons perform surgery because they have been trained to do so and because "they have always done it this way" or because they simply do not know any better, and (2) surgeons are incentivized to perform surgical procedures for financial gain, for renown, or for both.[17] The Hippocratic oath, "Do no harm," has become an almost obsolete medical ethos. Sadly, the ultimate medical utopia includes a transparent culture and a shared decision-making partnership between surgeons and patients for optimal health is but a dream.

Another study, done in 2016, surveyed hospital medical complications; the results found that one in six patients (16.8 percent) developed complications while in the hospital. It also found that one in 35 of those patients (2.8 percent) subsequently died without leaving the hospital. Based on a seven-day sample period, it estimated that, over a period of twelve months, 50 million hospital patients suffered complications following surgery and over 1.5 million died from those complications.[18]

DEATH BY MEDICINE

The 2014 video article entitled *Death by Medicine*, which comes from mercola.com, accurately describes the perils of conventional medicine in treating disease.[19] The video article was a wake-up call for me in my medical career. It inspired me to pursue epigenetics. I need to include the whole video article, verbatim. I do not feel that I could present it any better than how it was presented.

> *Conventional medicine has emerged as the leading cause of death and injury in the United States. Instead of lifting people's level of well-being, the American medical system is now doing more harm than good. Hospitals, which are supposed to be a haven for the ill, are plagued with medical malpractice and errors. In 1999, up to 100,000 people every year were at risk of dying from mistakes made in the hospital. Ten years later, that number rose to 180,000. Today that number could be as high as 440,000 casualties because of medical errors! Hospitals are also notorious breeding grounds for infections. Every day, one in twenty-five patients in the United States gets at least one infection associated with his or her hospital stay. Nearly two million people acquire a hospital infection every year, resulting in 90,000 deaths. The most common infections acquired in hospitals are pneumonia, surgical site infections, urinary tract infections, and bloodstream infections. But the most alarming are infections brought on by antibiotic-resistant bacteria. Antibiotic-resistant infections affect more than two million Americans every year, killing about 23,000 and accounting for a staggering $20 billion in annual direct health care costs.*
>
> *The conventional medical system has also transformed the United States into a drug-dependent nation. Nearly 70 percent of all Americans are taking at least one prescription drug for a chronic medical condition.*

Antibiotics, anti-depressants, and opioids top the list. One in five Americans takes at least one psychiatric medication. One in four senior citizens takes ten to nineteen pills a day and fills over thirty different prescriptions a year, if you add in drugs prescribed for other chronic senior conditions, such as gastroesophageal reflux disease (GERD), angina, depression, rheumatoid arthritis, and congestive heart failure, which could easily add up to two dozen or more drugs a day!

Children, too, are over-treated with medications and vaccines. In fact, they are the leading growth demographic for the drug industry. This growing dependency on drugs is not only putting our health on the line but also is placing a huge financial burden on our shoulders. In 2012, the United States led the world with $328.2 billion spent on prescription drugs. By 2017, those numbers are projected to be from $350 million to $380 billion. Who is making money off our so-called need for so many pharmaceuticals? Think about it—the market for pharmaceuticals and biotech drugs was projected to hit $1 trillion in 2014 and to rise to $1.2 trillion by 2017.

It is this excessive reliance on medications improving our quality of health? Not at all. Americans spend more on health care than any other industrialized nation, yet our country is not notably superior to any of the twelve comparable nations. Fifteen thousand people die every year in the United States from overdoses of opioids or narcotic pain pills. Between 1999 and 2010, the number of women who died from pain pill overdoses increased by a staggering 400 percent!

Even more disturbing is that studies of new drugs introduced from the mid-1970s through the mid-1990s show that only 11 percent-15.6 percent provide any therapeutic gain. More than one-third of the drugs were approved based on a single trial, without replication. Many other trials were small, short, and focused on laboratory values, or some other surrogate metric of effect, rather than clinical endpoints such as death.

Even the younger generation is now falling victim to the perils of this system. In a recent study of twenty-nine economically advanced countries, the United States ranked twenty-sixth in child well-being.

Out of twenty-nine developed countries, the United States is twenty-sixth in infant mortality, just ahead of Slovakia, Latvia, and Romania, which are the ONLY countries with infant mortality rates higher than six per 1,000 births. Among twenty-nine developed countries, the United States surpasses all in having the largest percentage of children aged eleven, thirteen, and fifteen who are overweight—a trend that predisposes them to chronic diseases as they grow up. These numbers reflect a health emergency in America.

"It is time for you to act now—stop bombarding your body with medical interventions that only put you in harm's way. Instead, reward yourself with the fit and lean body that comes from clean and healthy lifestyle habits. It is time to take control of your health!

THE PLACEBO EFFECT

During World War II, Henry Beecher, MD, was a pioneering American anesthesiologist, a medical ethicist, and an investigator of the placebo effect at Harvard Medical School.[20] The placebo effect is defined as the benefit produced by an inactive or a sham treatment, such as sterile water, a saline solution, or a sugar pill.[21] The placebo effect can be verbally induced or can result from the conditioning and the prior experiences that shape patient expectations.[22] The effect most likely stems from the patient's positive beliefs and from the expectations from, as well as from the positive interactions, with the doctor, in any treatment.

For millennia, the idea that your brain's positive beliefs can stimulate healing was already in practice in various ancient healing traditions. Your beliefs can convince your body that fake treatment is the real thing. This optimistic expectation of treatment will stimulate your own body's chemistry to cause beneficial physiological effects higher than what medication might have done. For example, patients may report pain relief after taking a placebo or a fake pill that looks like the same pain medication previously effective in easing the pain. Whenever the same stimulus is encountered in the future, patients condition themselves by shaping expectations, and they show responses that were previously imprinted in their memory. Learning and adaptation, therefore, drive a conditioned response.[22] It is epigenetics at work.

In 1961, the *nocebo* effect was recognized. It is the opposite of the placebo effect. The nocebo effect is activated by patients' negative expectations of treatment and unpleasant interactions with their doctors. Patients experience negative symptoms because they expect them. Patients have been known to manifest the side effects of a treatment, which could include vomiting, pain, headaches, even death[23] because patients have convinced themselves that the adverse effects will happen to them.

For the past twenty years, scientists have investigated how the placebo effect and the nocebo effect works in the human brain.[22] Both effects have the same mechanisms, which presumably are psychological, yet they can induce measurable changes in the body.[24] These scientists have developed scientific tools to study the mechanisms of the placebo effect and of the nocebo effect directly. They found that a placebo can cause the brain to release more opioids, a brain chemical released to the body to relieve pain and anxiety. The minimum threshold for placebo effect efficacy compared to any medication treatments is estimated between 30 percent to 40 percent.[25] Now let us compare the placebo effect with the drug efficacy. Starting in the mid-1970s, the federal government lowered the effectiveness standards for medications. Pharmaceutical companies were not required to prove full effectiveness. The effectiveness was dramatically reduced to somewhere between 11 percent and 15.6 percent.[26] This dramatic reduction was as if the passing grade for exams was lowered to somewhere between 11 percent and 15.6 percent.

The main priority of the pharmaceutical companies was to make sure that their drugs did not kill anyone right away.

Moderate-to-complete treatment success was no longer necessarily the goal post. Allen Roses, MD, the worldwide vice president of genetics at GlaxoSmithKline, stated in a December 2003 publication, *"The vast majority of drugs—more than 90%—only work in 30 percent or 50 percent of the people."* The statement means that most medications have only between a 30 percent chance and a 50 percent chance of working on the people taking them. How are these medications better than placebo pills?

To make matters worse, we have casually accepted the adverse consequences of medications, which may damage your internal organs, such as your liver and your kidneys. This is the main reason why your blood work must be monitored monthly when you are taking prescription medications. Your blood work is monitored primarily to check your liver and kidney poisoning levels from medications, not necessarily because your illness is healing. The reversal of chronic degenerative diseases is not the first goal when you are taking medications. Medications are used only for the relief of symptoms, without addressing their cause. Sadly, prolonged use of medications to control your symptoms is more profitable for the medical industry. A quick and sure cure for a disease is terrible for business.

Logically, let us step back and think about it. Take high blood pressure or hypertension, for example. Once you are diagnosed with hypertension, your doctor will start you on a hypertension medication right away. Your epigenetics risk factors are not even addressed, like hydration, sleep, healthy diet, and stress. (I will explain more about these factors in the latter part of the book.) Over time, if your hypertension persists, your doctor will continue adjusting your medication dose to keep your blood pressure artificially low. Rest assured that you still have uncorrected hypertension and that it is still causing havoc in your kidneys or your liver, whichever gives out first. Your high blood pressure is just artificially controlled with your medication, not reversed or cured.

Medication is suitable for only short-term use. Eventually, over time, at least two-to-five years, the secondary degenerative disease will be expected to set in from the adverse effects of prolonged use of medication. Such disease is an unfortunate consequence of hypertension, which is not addressed or reversed. Recent studies have shown that some of the common drugs used to treat high blood pressure can increase the risk of falls and fractures in older adults.[27,28] Once older adults fall and fracture their hips, they will spiral downhill, which can lead to early death.[28] These hypertension drugs are important for reducing the risk of heart attack and stroke. But, to prevent falls, as an older adult, you should consider the potential harms versus the benefits of antihypertensive medications cautiously when you first start them.

POLYPHARMACY SYNDROME

Polypharmacy syndrome is a twenty-first century epidemic. The syndrome is defined as the use of multiple drugs or the use of more drugs than are medically necessary. For this definition, medications that are not indicated, that are not effective, or that constitute a therapeutic duplication would be considered polypharmacy.[29] Many studies in ambulatory care define polypharmacy as taking five or more medications.[30]

Worldwide, it is a growing concern that most older adults take more than five-to-eight prescribed medications per day, with an unknown number of over-the-counter (OTC) supplements. International research shows that polypharmacy is common in older adults, with the highest number of drugs taken by residents in nursing homes. Nearly 50 percent of older adults take one or more medications that are not medically necessary.[30]

Polypharmacy syndrome is a severe medical condition that comes from multiple drug toxicity or from adverse drug effects that negatively affect multiple organs in your body, like your liver, your kidneys, and your brain. Research has clearly shown substantial evidence in the relationship between polypharmacy and negative clinical consequences. Very little rigorous research has been conducted on reducing unnecessary medications in frail, older adults, or patients approaching the end of life.[31] Sadly, there are no known long-term scientific studies on drug-to-drug interactions on patients who take two or more prescribed drugs daily, together with cheap OTC supplements.

In 2005, it was estimated that over 4.3 million health care visits were due to adverse drug effects.[32] The current medical-practice guidelines often require multiple medications to treat each chronic disease for optimal clinical benefit. In a population-based study, outpatients taking five or more medications had an 88 percent increased risk of experiencing an adverse drug effect, compared to those who were taking fewer medications.[33] Ironically, you are 88 percent guaranteed to be sick on the medicines that are supposed to help you. This is madness!

Patients are not aware that these medications bring more medical problems than they started with. Unfortunately, there are many negative consequences associated with polypharmacy. As expected, the common drugs that are guilty of adverse drug effects include anticoagulants, NSAIDs, cardiovascular medications, diuretics, antibiotics, anticonvulsants, benzodiazepines, and hypoglycemic medications.[34]

This is the kicker. According to a 2013 study, you have an 80 percent chance of damaging your liver from drug-to-drug interactions if you take five or more prescribed medications daily. Your probability risk will increase to 100 percent if you take twenty or more prescribed medications daily.[35] The compounding adverse effects of drug-to-drug interactions from all the prescribed drugs may result in a toxic liver, toxic kidneys, a toxic brain, and even death.

Multiple studies have validated the adverse clinical consequences of severe polypharmacy syndromes. They include increased functional declines, like diminished activities of daily living (ADL) abilities,[36] cognitive impairment, both delirium and dementia,[37] malnourishment,[38] and urinary incontinence.[39] Also, there is an increase in falls from certain medications. Sadly, falls are the main culprit for increased morbidity and increased mortality in older adults.[40]

It is difficult to diagnose the signs and symptoms of polypharmacy or overmedications at any age. They can mimic other mental or physical health conditions—often resulting in another prescription—or even the original problem for which they were prescribed. Diagnosis becomes even more challenging when polypharmacy is involved. When you see the list of symptoms below, these are suffered by almost 80 percent of the physical therapy patients I see in my practice. Endless clinical symptoms are unpredictable because of potential drug-to-drug interactions.[41]

So, what are the common signs and symptoms of polypharmacy or overmedications?

1. Fatigue, loss of energy
2. Abdominal pain
3. Bodily aches and pain
4. Motor and coordination problems
5. Falls and accidents
6. Frequent skin flushing and rashes
7. Unexplained weight loss or gain
8. Dramatic changes in mood
9. Lack of personal hygiene
10. Difficulty concentrating
11. Memory impairment
12. Mental cloudiness or confusion
13. Delayed thought process
14. Impaired rational thought
15. Hallucinations, delusions, and psychosis
16. Withdrawal symptoms when not using

When is enough, enough? And when is enough too much? We need to do a better job, especially with our older patients. Patients should be informed about the dangers of prolonged medication use, polypharmacy syndromes, and the importance of their body's self-healing mechanisms. They should also be informed about what behaviors cause these illnesses in the first place. More than ever, we need to use food as medicine—to provide our bodies with the raw materials for complete healing, with adequately prepared, nutrient-dense food, healthy beliefs, and coping mechanisms in the right environment. Patients need to be fully supported with proper information about what sustains a healthy body.

ALLOPATHIC MEDICINE VS. HOMEOPATHIC OR HOLISTIC MEDICINE

There are two main approaches to medicine that are practiced today: allopathic medicine and holistic or homeopathic medicine, also known as alternative medicine. Sadly, conventional Western medicine practices only allopathic medicine. It uses active chemical agents and physical interventions to treat or to suppress symptoms and the pathophysiologic processes of diseases or conditions. It is a reductionist process, focusing on the smaller problem or the symptoms, not the cause. It treats the body as separate, disconnected parts.

The allopathic approach used by the American health care system is reactive, focused only on the clinical symptoms, not on the root cause. It is a disease-oriented model of medicine. I called this "sick medical care." In contrast, the holistic or homeopathic approach to medicine looks at an individual's overall physical, mental, spiritual, and emotional well-being as part of the comprehensive treatment process. Holistic medicine focuses on the whole system or on the entire body, and it aims to be preventative. This is ideally what health care should be!

The main difference between allopathic care and holistic care is that standard medical care is about pure pharmaceuticals, medical procedures, and surgeries, while comprehensive health care focuses on nutritional and healthy lifestyle interventions. In reality, you can choose between medical care or health care.

A 1997 study estimates that, annually, more than 1 million patients are injured while in the hospital and that approximately 180,000 die because of these injuries. Furthermore, legally prescribed drug-related morbidity and mortality are common and are estimated to cost more than $136 billion a year.[42]

Modern Western medicine thrives on consensus data. Wherever the relevant consensus is at a given point is the driver of contemporary medicine. The problem with this system is that consensus can be artificially manipulated by the people who have the most to profit. And, of course, they will usually dominate the consensus. Western medicine is in danger of losing its integrity and intellectual independence from the almighty dollar. Sadly, profit trumps efficacy. I may be in trouble for saying that in recent years, Western medicine has not been designed for healing economically, efficiently, or most effectively. After more than thirty years of practicing in health care, I can honestly say that most health care providers are acutely aware of this fact. It is sad.

Sadly, standard Western medical care relies heavily on surgeries, prescription pills, and the infamous twelve-minute doctor visit. According to the CDC, in 2010, 92.4 percent of U.S. surgeries were deemed unnecessary and unsuccessful.[43] It is documented that more deaths are due to overdose and overuse of prescribed medicines than deaths by any diseases or epidemics combined yearly.[44]

Real health care should focus on prevention, reversal, and maintenance. It should guarantee a better quality of life, compared to what standard Western medicine sick care guarantees. Epigenetics is incorporated into holistic health care. It is beyond just eating healthy and having a healthy lifestyle. It is all the factors together that modify your immune system and gene expression.

Death is not preventable. The quality of the way you live and die matters. Ideally, one is supposed to die during old age, naturally and peacefully (with exceptions for traumatic incidents). Everyone should leave the earth with dignity, surrounded by family at home, not with the slow death from prolonged, heavy use of medications and with frequent visits to the impersonal and sterile environment of a hospital. As a physical therapist, I cannot say enough that you are supposed to have a good quality of life without chronic pain or degenerative disease.

Modern medicine is only approximately 200 years old. The arrogance of Western medicine's superiority over all other ancient healing traditions is a tragedy. It is an incomplete, but evolving, growth of knowledge. Indeed, it has advanced the medical interventions in acute and traumatic injuries, but not in the prevention and reversal of degenerative diseases. Both ways of healing have their place in human health. We need both, and we can learn from both approaches. They are complementary to each other. Allopathic medicine and holistic medicine are the two halves in the practice of human health.

Historically, the practice of modern medicine was taught in a more balanced curriculum, in both holistic and allopathic methods, in all 200 American medical schools. Until around the 1930s, naturopathic medicine gradually declined, almost to the point of extinction because of biomedical opposition and the advent of miracle drugs. From 1940 to 1963, the American Medical Association (AMA) fought against any natural-based or nonpharmaceutical-based medical systems.[45] Modern medicine lost its holistic half and was directed toward a solely chemical path. Sadly, allopathic medicine is now the only standard of advanced medical care. Fortunately, there is a recent revival of holistic medicine. I am very optimistic that I will see both practices of medicine jointly appreciated and studied again.

SICK MEDICAL CARE FOR PROFIT

The business paradigm for today's health care is profit first, then treating people's symptoms. Optimal health and 'the cure' are not primary health care goals. There is more money in prolonging a disease than preventing it. Our health care system is designed primarily for profit and to maintain sickness, not to cure it.

Take, for example, the medical evolution of therapy for Type 1 and Type 2 diabetes. In 1922, a young Canadian surgeon named Frederick Banting, MD, discovered insulin. It was the most significant medical breakthrough for preventing children with Type 1 diabetes from dying. At that time, most children diagnosed with diabetes were expected to die within a year. Dr. Banting and his colleagues intentionally did not patent their insulin invention for the most altruistic reason. On January 23, 1923, Dr. Banting, Dr. Collip, and Dr. Best were awarded U.S. patents on insulin and the method used to make it. They all sold these patents to the University of Toronto for $1 each to benefit humanity! Later that year, Dr. Banting and Dr. Macleod were awarded the Nobel Prize in medicine for the discovery of insulin.

Before the discovery of insulin in 1922, Type 2 diabetes was reversed entirely in six-to-eight weeks with a diet consisting mainly of fat and protein, with the much-reduced amount of carbohydrates needed to sustain life.[46] With a short-term dietary sacrifice, this new diet completely reversed Type 2 diabetes. Initially, externally manufactured insulin was not for the treatment of Type 2 diabetes.

Unfortunately, the current diabetic protocol for Type 2 diabetes has completely changed its trajectory. It is no longer working toward a complete cure for the disease but for controlling its symptoms. By prolonging the disease, the health care industry giants are positioned to make more money by controlling Type 2 diabetes with medications, according to conventional Western medicine throughout the patient's lifespan. According to the American Diabetes Association, people with diagnosed diabetes incur average medical expenditures of $16,752.00 per year, of which about $9,601.00 is attributed to diabetes. On average, people with diagnosed diabetes have medical costs approximately 2.3 times higher than what expenditures would have been in the absence of diabetes.[47] The average person with diabetes will live twenty to thirty years with conventional medical intervention. Let us do the math: $17,000.00 × twenty years = $3.4 million, as compared to curing the disease with a strict diet that might cost an average of $3,000.00 at the most!

Besides, it is sad to note that all medical schools teach only the study of medications, not nutrition or epigenetics. It is estimated that most medical schools teach a total of about two hours of nutritional courses although, I hear the medical schools are changing their number of courses. Sadly, it will not be soon enough for most patients. Most practitioners automatically prescribe diabetic medications. Eventually, they will refer diabetic patients to a conventional dietician, who may design a dietary program containing processed food. It may not be the optimal nutrition for a diabetic patient who is hoping for a cure.

This is also dismally true in my physical therapy business. If I help heal my patients effectively in less time than the average physical therapist (PT), I get paid less. I get paid per session, not for efficacy. It is the main reason why I left my previous job and decided to open my own holistic PT clinic almost seven years ago.

For almost eight years, I was the clinical director of a busy outpatient PT clinic. We saw thirty to fifty patients per day. We were very successful in helping patients feel better. But, one day, the practice owner talked to the entire staff of the PT department and told us that we are not making more money, even though we are one of the best PT clinics in the area. She adamantly emphasized the problem—we were not making money like other PT clinics in the area because we fixed the patients to pain-free too soon. She proceeded to inform us that we had the shortest or the least PT visits, thus affecting our clinic revenues. Her speech to us did not sit well with my core being as a PT, so I decided it was time to quit. The owner and I had hit the fork in the road. Her sole mission was for profit at any cost, while I was still holding onto my altruistic ideals. The next day, I came to work and submitted my resignation. After eight months, I was able to open the Holistic Physical Therapy Clinic. I must admit that she was right. It was not a money-making business to help patients effectively. However, like the little train caboose, the Holistic Physical Therapy Clinic has been trying very hard to strike a balance between healing and sustainability. The rest is history.

 In epigenetics, your gene expression is 100 percent within your control.

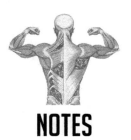

NOTES

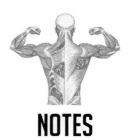

NOTES

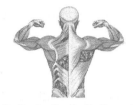

CHAPTER 2

THE ART OF HOLISTIC HEALING

"The human body, when functioning well, is pain-free. It is an intelligent, self-healing organism. Any pain and diseases are earned. Essentially, your body is dependent on healthy food, optimal hydration, consistent detox, restorative sleep, proper exercise, a happy heart, and a peaceful soul."
—Dr. Gigi Siton, DPT

HOLISTIC HEALING 101

The healthy human body is made perfect and free of chronic pain.

Your body does not have the jargon of medical diagnosis that modern medicine uses. It just knows that something is not working when it lacks the raw materials to maintain and repair itself. When it is healthy, it is free of unresolved pain and disease. However, when something is not working right in your body, it will try to communicate with you in many efficient ways. The primary default system of your body, when it detects anomaly or threat, is pain. We need to change how we address pain.

Pain is a friend.
Pain is your friend. It is your loyal and handy messenger. This idea contradicts what I was taught in PT school. I was taught that pain was public enemy number one, not the body's loyal messenger. Pain lets you know when something is not working right and when that something needs your attention.

Pain receptors, also called nociceptors, are a group of sensory neurons with specialized nerve endings widely distributed in the skin, in the deep tissues (including the muscles and the joints), and in most of the internal organs.[48] They react to injury or potentially harmful stimuli by transmitting painful messages first to the nerve endings via the spinal cord and finally to the brain. For the sake of this book, I will refer to nociceptors as pain sensors.

Pain can come from any part of your body. Physical pain, emotional pain, and spiritual pain can come from different sources. It has been known that emotional pain and spiritual pain will ultimately present themselves as physical pain.

Pain is psychoemotional.
It is about time to address the emotional layer of pain. When I was in PT school, if physical therapy interventions did not work with certain patients, we were made to believe that they must be faking the pain. Sadly, the faking was called "malingering syndrome." I used to resent treating these patients. Back then, I was not aware of the powerful connection between your body and your emotions.

Fortunately, science has finally caught up with the studies validating the powerful connection between your body and trauma. It is high time we incorporate the significant role of your belief system in the healing of your biology. Your body retains memory from physical or emotional trauma. If it is not addressed correctly, intense emotional stress from any traumatic experience will leave a mark on specific organs of your body.

In 1985, the Barral Institute was established, an international health education, training, and research organization dedicated to the advancement and validation of the therapeutic effects of Visceral Manipulation, Nerve Manipulation, and related Manual Therapies. According to the Barral Institute, the human body is the seat of an emotion-organ-behavior-organ cycle. Intense stress is imprinted into your brain, and your brain will transmit excess pressure onto your organs, whose fibrous matter immediately records the emotion. It is how psychosomatic reactions begin.

Each organ will retain specific emotions. When we experience painful emotions, our feet or hands may not be in pain, but our organs are very receptive to our negative or positive emotions and feelings. The pain memory of our organs is massively dependent on the emotional intensity, the severity, and the duration of the stress we experience. According to Jean-Pierre Barral, DO, MRO (F), RPT, in his book *The Messages of the Body*, each person has weak organ links, possibly because of a genetic predisposition or an unhealthy lifestyle. The fragile link organ could be vulnerable and could become the leading site for stress retention.[49]

Occasionally, some physical pain is coming from an emotional upset, which then negatively affects the associated organ.[50] Conversely, when an organ is physically damaged, it can induce psychological symptoms to surface. All people have different behavioral reactions and emotional symptoms in stressful situations.

Understanding the emotional connection with our organs is crucial in our healing and in maintaining optimal well-being. Our well-being is dependent on our effective coping mechanism. When one of our physical problems is resolved, our behavioral and emotional state will improve, as well. By the same token, as our behavior and our emotions improve, our physical symptoms will also improve.[49]

Jean Pierre Barral, DO, in his book *Understanding the Messages of Your Body,* indicated that your liver retains anger and bad memories. Your pancreas retains social stress, a death that you have not accepted, or a childhood that has been crushed or stolen. Your gallbladder retains a constant preoccupation and worry and fear of conflict. Your heart retains guilt, hatred, and fear of dying, while low back pain, especially in men, retains intense financial stress.

A classic example is Post-Traumatic Stress Disorder (PTSD). It happens after car wrecks, after head concussions, after extreme emotional stress, or after war trauma. Most patients who suffer from this disorder will present both physical and emotional distress. We must address healing both heart and mind, systematically.

In 2017, a study was conducted with post-concussion syndrome patients describing the effects of Craniosacral Therapy (CST), Visceral Manipulation (VM), and Neural Manipulation (NM) modalities as treatments. The patients included eleven male retired professional football players from the National Football League and the Canadian Football League who had been medically diagnosed with post-concussion syndrome. After ten two-hour sessions, twice a day, the treatments resulted in statistically significant improvements in concussed patients' pain intensity, range of motion (ROM), memory, cognition, and sleep.[51]

With my psychology background, I feel fortunate in my practice to appreciate the emotional factor of my patients' suffering. I can intuitively identify the additional emotional layer of their physical pain. I have seen this phenomenon in my patients with pelvic floor pain, as well as some patients with neck pain and back pain.

I have seen these cases many times in my clinic. About 60 to 70 percent of my patients do not suffer from pure physical pain. The majority of my patients suffer from emotional stress. They come with emotional burdens alongside their physical symptoms. Not all pain is physically caused. In these situations, I use craniosacral intervention, combined with a consultation with a life coach, if the patient is open to the idea. Once patients become emotionally stable, their physical pain is easy to resolve with holistic physical therapy interventions.

Pain is a time traveler.

In the previous paragraphs, we learned how your body remembers trauma. In this section, I am going to discuss the unconscious verbalization of past pain trauma as if it had just happened. I call it a pain-memory slip or pain-time traveler. I define it as a memory of past traumatic pain in the body spilling into present physiological sensations. It is the presentation of the ongoing physiologic response of trauma that happened in the past. It is an unresolved pain that made a permanent scar on a person's psyche. The origin may be an emotional injury or an actual physical harm, like rape, being in a war, or even in a car accident, and the like. All of which are hallmarks of Post-Traumatic Stress Disorder (PTSD), in one degree or another.

Let me give you an example in my practice. During my first consultation with new patients, I always try to investigate a thorough pain history and to understand why they seek physical therapy. I listen very carefully to each patient. Most of my patients who have had mild-to-severe PTSD will unconsciously use the present tense in describing the traumatic event that happened in the past. It does not matter if it happened when they were six years old, thirteen years old, or even just a few years ago. I think that their minds and their bodies are unconsciously suspended at that traumatic moment every time they think or talk about it. Their bodies will produce the same physiologic responses as if the traumatic event had just happened, even though they are only talking about the trauma. It is almost like experiencing the same pain and injury repeatedly. The event happened maybe once, but their minds and bodies seem to hash it over and over again.

I can spot this pain-memory-slip phenomenon in most of my patients. Once they are made aware of it, fortunately, the mild cases tend to be able to resolve on their own. However, for moderate to severe cases, my patients must seek more professional emotional help to fix it. Once their memory of pain is in its proper conscious place in the past, their recovery is much more linear and straightforward.

Pain is for protection.
The first layer of your protection system is your pain sensors. Necessarily, your pain sensors are present in every cell of your body. Some areas have a higher concentration of pain sensors than others. Pain sensitivity differs according to the number of pain sensors or receptors in an area. The main job of pain is the protection of vital organs and tissues from damage. Pain is your body's first responder for repairing injury.

Your feet and your hands are very efficient in detecting touch and pain. Your gut has more pain sensors than your brain and spinal cord combined. Your rib cage has many pain sensors for the protection of your critical internal organs. Anybody who has suffered either rib dislocation or rib fracture knows the extreme agony of rib pain in any position—even with a tiny expansion of the rib cage, like breathing.

The grand central station for warning of pain is located in your brain. Your body processes the pain sensation and activates the necessary response back to the tissues where pain sensors are located. It is designed to have an efficient automatic pain response process between them, wherein there is constant communication between your cells, locally, and your brain, centrally.

In an injury scenario, pain is the first alarm signal to the brain. It will send messages to your brain by activating pain sensations specific to the affected area through a protein enzyme. This messenger protein enzyme will reach the brain and relay the signal to start the repair process. The brain will automatically respond by activating the acute inflammatory process around the affected areas. Once the affected cells have been repaired and healed, the local cells will stop sending the pain protein enzyme. Then, the pain goes away! If you have a well-functioning immune system, your body will be restored quickly when it is provided with the right raw materials like healthy good food, proper hydration, and a suitable healing environment, like rest and sound sleep.

Pain is the significant signal that your body uses as an immediate form of communication, just like the indicator light in your car when something is malfunctioning or when your gasoline is about to run out. Your body gives you subtle hints of pain; then your body gives you a whisper of pain, which gradually turns into intense pain. Finally, if the low-grade pain is ignored, it will stop you in your tracks, like a major heart attack or a degenerative disease. The disease starts when you regularly ignore pain. Chronic neurodegenerative diseases are usually the result of chronic neglect of the body.

Pain is your body's loyal and honest messenger.
Most people are not taught how to listen to these messages or signals. Conventional Western medicine is designed to shoot the messenger. It is geared to turn off the warning light or to stifle the pain-signal mechanism in your body instead of addressing the cause of your pain.

In my holistic PT practice, I always teach my patients that pain is your friend. It is there for you to honor and to act upon. It is interesting to note that when you honor pain by giving it what it needs, it will go away from you as soon as it comes. I usually encourage my patients to befriend their pain. I need to know of their pain to let me know whether or not the physical therapy is working. At the start of every physical therapy session, I and my colleagues ask the patients for their pain levels. Their answers give us a benchmark against which to measure their progress, and their answers tell us if our holistic PT protocol needs to be advanced or modified. If the holistic PT treatment works, the pain will stop without medications. I also encourage my patients not to be afraid of pain. If it ever comes back, it means that your body's alert mechanism is intact. In Dr. Fereydoon Batmanghelidj's book *Your Body's Cries for Water*, he writes that since your body is 75 percent water, most of the time, the initial cause of your body's aches and pains is just unintended chronic dehydration. At this stage, it would be wise to try water and to rest before taking medications. I will discuss more on hydration in Book Three.

Most chronic pain and chronic diseases are acquired.
Most chronic degenerative diseases are self-inflicted. In other words, you have inflicted such diseases to your body over time. The excellent news is that they are fixable! My patients always blame old age for their pain. And when we resolve their problem with a holistic PT approach, they are surprised that the pain is gone. It has nothing to do with age!

Modern medicine has convinced many people to accept pain and medications as a natural part of aging. I do not agree. I have seen ninety-year-old patients who can do push-ups and who can perform all the therapy exercises in the clinic pain-free, once they are better. I also see patients as young as eight years old in constant pain because of joint arthritis and Type 2 diabetes, as a result of a poor diet, coupled with a sedentary lifestyle. Aging gracefully and pain-free is how your body normally functions.

I was a pediatric physical therapist for nearly six years. Play is a physiological need for the body and the brain to be strong and healthy. Tragically, most children no longer play outside to get much-needed vitamin D3 through sunshine, to improve their joint health, their body balance, and their brain coordination. Television and video games have taken over outdoor play. Playing with one or more children is the most interactive game one can play. It is a great way to learn cooperation and emotional connections. If you laugh, the children laugh back, and if you hit them, they might hit you back, or they cry. One learns to negotiate on how to get along. It is a pure, simple joy to play outside. Playing outside is not just for kids, either. Swinging on a swing at the playground for at least twenty minutes a day improves muscle tone and attention span, as well as vestibular sense and balance. Play is also a form of exercise that increases the body's muscles' capacity to absorb insulin efficiently. Hanging on the monkey bars improves reading and upright posture, not to mention strengthening your upper core muscles and the cartilage in your shoulder, elbow, and wrist joints. I incorporate hanging on the bars as an essential rehabilitation skill for all patients with rotator cuff injuries.

In addition, playing in the dirt improves our immune system.[52] According to the hygiene hypothesis, the microbes and their products have an essential role in human immune system regulation. The hygiene hypothesis has been a topic of contention ever since the term was first coined in 1989 by an epidemiologist, Dr. David P Strachan, MD.[53] It proposes that a cause of the recent rapid rise in allergic disorders could be a lower incidence of infection in early childhood.[54] When one defensive system lacks practice, perhaps from an overly sanitary lifestyle, the other system becomes too powerful and overreacts to harmless substances like pollen.[55] You are less likely to develop allergies and asthma if you have been exposed to microbes as a child from your siblings, from your pets, and from playing outside in the dirt.

Self-healing is an inherent automatic process.
Your body is inherently designed for your health, preprogrammed to self-heal. It's an intelligent machine! Your body's healing process is automatic. It functions for health. A disease is an expression of

a malfunctioning healing process. Your body does not wait for you to tell it what to heal first. It works 24/7 to maintain your optimal health. From conception, cell division is well organized and inherently synchronized on what develops first to make you a fully functional human being. Your body knows what is not working, as well as when and how to fix what is not working. It can detect malfunctions and compensates itself until it is in order again. Your body has all the bells and whistles to communicate what it needs and what is going on. We just do not want to listen, or we are not taught how to listen and how to interpret the body's messages and signals. The problem arises when we get in the way of the standard and efficient healing process.

Be kind to your body.
We need to start to be the kindest person our bodies ever met. I always tell my patients that when you love a person, you will take extra care of that person, to make sure he or she is well-loved and well taken-care of. Let us start that with ourselves—not in a narcissistic way but in a kind and loving way. It is guaranteed that your body will provide the best shape you need to perform at the optimal level, once your body is healthy. Olympic champions and elite athletes always invest in healthy food and lifestyles to achieve optimal performance. You don't need to be an Olympian to achieve unlimited success. Unlimited success starts when you learn how to be kind to yourself and when you listen to your body.

Your body's healing has a sacred pace.
I always get asked this question: how long will it take to return to normal? I always respond that your body heals itself. It has its own sacred pace to restore God's masterpiece! You are being stitched back together one cell at a time. Only your body's own healing process and its sacred pace know when it will be healed, as well as how long it will take. You must support it. You must be aware

that the healing process will take time. Medicine is an imperfect science; it has an estimated healing period, but ultimately, your body's healing happens according to the proper environment and the suitable raw materials you provided it.

Again, I cannot emphasize it enough. Your only job is to provide the right raw materials and the right environment for your body to heal. Many of my patients would like to put a hard deadline on the healing so they can mark it on their busy calendars. Most of the time, when I respond with a ballpark period, I get this answer, "I do not have time!" Worse, their doctors tell my patients that there is a shorter period for their bodies to heal. My patients then inform me, purposefully, about the deadline given them by their doctors to make sure I adhere to it. The time frame for healing is also a typical Medicare patients' dilemma in the clinic. Medicare has limited them to ten to twelve visits, which is three to four weeks of extensive physical therapy. However, a full recovery, with post-surgery rehab, will take an average range of six months to two years if my patients are entirely devoted to healing, with the best epigenetics support.

You are the only person who can assist your healing process, not your medical doctor. He is not the person who heals you, but he can guide you. He is your body's translator for Western medicine, or, if you choose alternative medicine, you have an alternative medicine translator. The healing process inside your body does not change, whichever school of medicine you have chosen.

I agree with Dr. Alec Burton, DO, PhD, about his healing paradigm. He was a founding member and past president of the International Association of Hygienic Physicians, Inc. USA, a specialist's organization of primary care doctors working with fasting and lifestyle management. According to him, *"Healing is a biological/living process ... It's inherent in the organism! We have no control over the human body's processes. There's no such person as a healer. There's no such thing as a healing agent or cure. There's no such thing as a chemical, a drug, food, or any other ingredient that will take the place of the living processes of life. All healing is self-healing. It is not something that somebody else does to you. It's something you do for yourself."*

The whole irony of the healing process is that the more you rush the healing process, the longer it takes. Patience and kindness are also an integral part of healing, along with the best epigenetics interventions. Most patients are rushing and don't take care of themselves. They look at me as if healing is my job, not theirs. I quickly remind them that I am just a teacher and a coach to guide them through their recovery. I am trained to interpret body signs and messages—hence my physical therapy training. But 90 percent of the work comes from and is done by them. Physical therapy breaks down the stages and the steps for achieving maximum healing. It is supervised training, with an expert eye to guide the healing process.

Brain setting for healing.
Another important factor in healing is tuning to the right-brain setting for that process. You have two autonomic nervous system modes in your brain: the parasympathetic mode and the sympathetic mode. The parasympathetic mode is the healing setting. It is the ideal *rest-and-relax* setting, while the sympathetic mode is the *fight-or-flight* setting. Stress is a sympathetic mode that will prevent healing because it compromises your immune system. We will discuss more on this topic in the Autonomic Nervous System section in Book Two.

Overthinking your healing process is not helpful. Most patients overthink the process. They think that they are in control of the healing process, rushing the timeline. They want the magic bullet, fast! My consistent response is that the healing process is not instant, and that is how your body is divinely designed. Your body will heal one cell at a time, according to its sacred pace; just do not get in its way!

On the other side of the spectrum, some of my patients get very defensive when I ask them for a more detailed history of their problem. I have had patients who have passively surrendered their recovery to their doctor, without questioning and informing themselves about the process. I have seen patients who have had nineteen nerve-block injections into their spines for severe chronic pain without permanent relief. The problem with nerve-block injections is that they *turn off* the pain signal, along with a specific distribution of the targeted nerve, without addressing the leading cause of the pain. They are only a temporary fix. They typically last one or two weeks and then wear off, as your body absorbs them.[56] In addition, the risks of nerve block injections can be severe, such as infections on the sites where the nerve-block injections are made, bleeding, accidental delivery of medication into the bloodstream, unexpected spread of drugs to other nerves, and hitting the *wrong* nerve in an attempt to block the targeted nerve. Besides, if fluoroscopy or computer tomography (CT) is used, there will be low-level radiation.[55]

Sadly, most of the time, the pain will come back vigorously. What I observed with my patients is that the intensity of pain is usually worse than their original pain level before the nerve-block injections, hence more injections! This vicious cycle of *pain-injection-pain* never ends, until someone wakes up. I have always suggested to my patients that, after three tries, if nerve-block injections do not work, maybe they should stop them. Otherwise, they become added insults to injury. They should seriously consider another treatment method.

To paraphrase Albert Einstein, my patients are performing the same actions while expecting different results—a classic definition of insanity. Most patients love their doctors and hate to disagree with them. In defense of most doctors, most of them try their best to provide proper care to their patients, according to their medical training. Generally, they mean no harm. The tragic thing about this perpetually failed medical treatment is that the patients believed that it was a good idea, even if it did not work for them. Their unquestioning faith and trust in their doctors are more robust than the efficacy of the treatment itself. Even the placebo effect failed them.

In my clinic, I usually tell my patients to let me give them two weeks of holistic PT treatments, and if they do not work, to let us regroup, to reassess and to try something else. At some point, each practitioner must know when to refer a patient to a different practitioner who can help better. My career is not about me. It is about helping patients to feel better and to restore their health. Practitioners of modern medicine have no incentive to heal patients efficiently because they are paid for procedures rendered, not for efficacy.

TEN CORE FOUNDATIONAL HEALING PRINCIPLES

1. *It is a divine intelligent design.*

Regarding this first healing principle, may I share the spiritual beliefs that shaped me and that helped me choose this noble medical profession? I must apologize ahead of time if you become offended by my Christian sensibility throughout this book. It comes from my thirty years of being a practiced clinician. The more in-depth studies in the medical sciences of healing I made, the deeper my spiritual realization became. My faith and my reason augment each other beautifully.

Healing is a divine design. It is God's given gift to humanity. The caveat is that you must use your God-given free will for healing to work. It means that you must choose to be healthy every time. Your body has an innate intelligent design to self-heal and to make new body parts. You are given an entire updated body approximately every two to seven years! It is almost as if God guarantees you as human beings to have an updated car every two years, given that you provide the right food that He made for your body. Healing also needs the right heart and the perfect environment for it to thrive. You are designed to thrive, not just to survive.

Here is one estimate on the natural regeneration of human body cells: your body can make a new liver cell in four-to-six weeks; a new pancreas cell in four-to-eight weeks; new blood cells in three months; new skin cells in six weeks; and a whole new body in eighteen months-to-seven years!

2. *Healing is as natural as breathing or farting!*
If you are breathing, you are healing. Breathing is vital in a person's survival. Five seconds without breathing oxygen, and a person will die instantly! The death of brain cells occurs almost immediately without oxygen, if there is a delay in medical intervention. It is very therapeutic to maintain proper breathing exercises to provide the lungs and the brain with a constant, fresh supply of much-needed oxygen. More on breathing in Book Three.

Farting is an essential bodily function, especially after surgery. Most nurses are aware of this essential function. In the surgical-recovery unit of any hospital, post-surgery protocol requires patients to pass good farts before they can be discharged. Such protocol shows that your digestive plumbing is in proper working condition to prevent gastrointestinal complications after you are discharged.

The different odors of farts could reveal something about your digestive system. Stomach gas is produced by fermentation of undigested food. It could mean that there are more harmful gut bacteria or pathogens causing bloating symptoms, usually after consumption of a meal. The stronger the smell is, the more harmful bacteria are in your gut. Ideally, there needs to be a healthy balance between the good bacteria and the harmful bacteria.[57] Generally, the amount of soluble and insoluble fiber content in your diet helps determine the healthy ratio between the good and the bad bacteria in your gut.

3. *Healing takes place at night.*
We are innately connected to the rhythm of the earth.[58] The body is programmed to heal only at night, when you are at full rest. God also made body parts that help with the healing process at night. Sleep has a critical restorative and healing function in the body. Most of our endocrine system function best at night, in the dark.[59]

Our hormones and neurotransmitters are efficiently manufactured in the digestive system. Primarily, the different endocrine glands will utilize the raw materials to produce hormones for use throughout the body. Most neurotransmitters are made in our digestive system for brain use.[60] For example, sleep has different stages. One of the hormones produced during sleep is melatonin. Its peak production happens only at night, during sleep. Melatonin is needed for weight loss and white blood cell production. There is strong evidence of a link between insufficient sleep and the risk of cancer. Studies have shown that most cancer patients have poor sleeping habits.[61] Likewise, most mental or psychological disorders, including schizophrenia and depression, will significantly improve if the patients have a good night's sleep.[62] It usually takes eight hours of sleep to recharge what your body used during the day. More on sleep in Book Three.

4. *Healing is intuitive.*
Healing is intuitive. *Intuition* is a gut sensation that serves as a subtle warning from instinctive feeling rather than from conscious reasoning. You need to honor and to be obedient to your body's signals. The mind and body connection are powerful. You need to master how to listen to your intuition. Your body signals your intuition first; then it signals through the different body sensations, such as tiredness, pain, and sleepiness.

Your body knows innately and prioritizes what is essential for survival. The primary survival organs are your heart, your lungs, and your brain. These organs must be maintained 24/7 for healthy functioning. When you feel tired, rest! Most people know, intuitively, what they need to heal, but they talk themselves out of it because they have so much to do. Your body does not need much to recover—just drinking enough water or taking power naps. Taking a power nap is like giving your body a little reboot during the day, and your body will function so much more efficiently. I am a big proponent of a midday nap. When I was growing up, my father took a long nap at midday. He was a lawyer and the dean at the College of Law in my hometown. Every day, he would come home from work to eat lunch at noon and then take a siesta until 1:30 p.m. He would feel recharged and refreshed before going back to work. Then, he would come home for dinner around 5:30 p.m. to eat supper with the family; then, he would go back to teach law until 10 p.m. He even taught classes at 6:00 a.m. on Saturdays. He was always full of energy and wore a big smile all the time. When I was in grade school, I used to hate siesta. I thought it was a waste of time. Now I need it. At my PT clinic, we turn down the lights at noon. We all lie down after lunch and try to rest. I always look forward to taking a twenty-minute power nap at noon as much as I can, so I will be recharged for the rest of the day.

5. *The fastest way to stimulate healing is fasting.*[63]

Just as we should sleep only when we feel tired, we should eat only when we feel hungry. When sick, fast. Fasting is defined as abstaining from eating. It has been practiced since ancient times. Many ancient religions have historically incorporated fasting in their practices. Consistent fasting is necessary to maintain good health.[64] Intuitively, humans must have realized very early on that taking a break from hunting and gathering, mostly eating, reboots one's spiritual, emotional, and physical well-being. Fasting allows more blood circulation to your brain, instead of the blood just being used to digest food.[65] It has been shown in studies that your hypothalamus and your pineal gland work best in a fasting state.[66,67]

There are many kinds of fasting. There is fasting from solid food (drinking only bone broth), fasting from all meat (eating only vegetables), fasting from all food (drinking only fresh juices), intermittent fasting, and the biblical fasting (drinking only water). These will be discussed later, in Book Three.

6. *Healing is holistic.*

Health and healing are holistic. There are seven ingredients to this interconnected integral healing relationship, namely: (1) proper nutrition and proper hydration; (2) restorative sleep; (3) a happy heart, meaning healthy relationships with self and others; (4) continuous intellectual growth; (5) an active spiritual connection; (6) proper exercise; and (7) consistent detox and fasting. All of these factors will be discussed throughout this book.

7. *Healing is a personal responsibility.*

Healing is a personal responsibility. It *is* your body, after all. The first step in healing is to choose to heal. Once you decide on healing and you prioritize it, it will set your immune system in that direction. In his book *Biology of Belief*, Bruce Lipton, PhD, indicates that your conscious decisions affect your overall biology, especially your healing process. Indeed, healing is automatic; however, your deliberate prioritization to heal causes the mind and the body to be in sync, which will positively support your immune system to move in the direction of healing.

In the book *Overcome Your Core Fears* by Mark F. Kialing, PsyD, I learned that harboring any inner doubts or fears will slow down any repairs and the rebuilding of your body. All the people's best healing efforts around you would not matter, even if they have the best intention for you to heal. Without your cooperation and willingness, healing will be less effective.

8. *Healing is also a team effort.*

The primary responsibility of your healing rests on your shoulders. In this light, healing must also be a team effort. It is best to create a sound healing team to support and to encourage your recovery. It starts with being kind to your spouse or your family as your healing partner. Having a good team supporting the whole healing process makes it a community effort. It will also give the people around you an opportunity to show how much they care for you. You can allow them to take care of you and to show you how much they love you. Most people find it easier to give love and attention than to receive it. In contrast, most people with illness are not comfortable receiving care and attention. Healing with a team around you is an excellent opportunity to savor the attention and the love that is performed for you. Studies have shown that when patients are alone, there is a higher mortality rate.[68]

9. *Fortify your gut; fortify your immune system.*

Your gut is the factory of your immune system. Your gut makes the components of all your immune system's needs. It supplies what is needed to make new body parts. What you eat or drink becomes your body parts or destroys your body parts. Whatever enters your mouth either heals you or harms you. There's no in-between. The quality of food in your diet will produce the same quality of your body parts. Your body cannot build new parts on fake foods or food-like substances. Any processed foods dampen bodily functions. Your body recognizes such foods as junk and toxic substances. The toxins deposited in your body burdens the system and stops ongoing healing and repair. Lousy food may even add insult to injury: it could also help create a disease process.

Your gut always needs a massive protective fortification, like castle walls—just as a castle fortress is made with massive stone walls so it can better withstand all kinds of assaults during a battle. Your gut needs fortification with the right type of foods, like fresh, organic vegetables and filtered healthy water, along with the right environment to battle disease and to rebuild your body. More on your gut in Book Three.

Hydration is very critical for survival and healing. Your blood consists of 80 percent water, and drinking filtered water infuses your blood and all your body cells. Depriving your body of essential water that it needs depletes your blood right away. Water can also flush toxins so that they do not stay in your body to cause problems. More on this topic in Book Three.

10. *Stay close to your ancestral diet.*
Your ancestral diet means an eating pattern according to your biogenetic origin. This style of eating will be healthiest when you eat the foods your body is best accustomed to. It is wise to stay as close to your ancestral diet as you can. Your body will be able to handle your trying new foods occasionally. However, switching entirely to a new diet that is far from your ancestral diet is likely to cause a metabolic upset. Eating a different diet over an extended period will cause chronic disease or could even lead to cancer.[69]

Your body follows the principle of bio-individuality. I learned this concept over a decade ago, during my postgraduate training with the Nutritional Therapy Association in Austin, Texas. It means that there is no "one-diet-fits-all," especially here in America. Each of you has a highly individualized metabolic requirement that is massively dependent on your genetic background, your physical size, your metabolic rate, your family, and your cultural background. You have your own set of ancestral biogenetics that has an inherently different metabolic response to food and your environment. Even though you or your ancestors have crossed the Pacific Ocean or the Atlantic Ocean, your gut has not completely deviated from its inherited genetic metabolism.

For example, as an Asian woman, I have lactose intolerance. Anthropologically, in Asian countries, cows were not native.

Consequently, I am missing the enzyme to digest a cow's lactose. I guess my Asian genes did not adapt to breaking down a cow's lactose into my gut because the lactose has not been in my ancestors' foods for a millennium. Because of my lactose intolerance, cow's milk gives me an upset stomach, and shooting diarrhea is guaranteed every time. It also gives me major dead-animal, stinky farts! Lactose intolerance is also common for Blacks and Hispanics. However, those of northern European descent can usually process cow's milk just fine.

Another case for bio-individuality: some people can be vegetarian, even vegan, and they do okay; some people cannot.[70] A vegetarian or vegan diet makes some people deficient in nutrients or makes them gain weight. In my clinic, we see vegan or vegetarian patients with severe symptoms of vitamin and mineral deficiency.[71] We test them individually for vitamin deficiencies or food intolerances and allergies. Eventually, they may require nutritional therapy to restore optimal health.

On the basis of my genetic background and the place where I grew up, I find that I can eat just 10 percent-to-20 percent of animal-based protein, preferably seafood (like fish) and vegetables. In the past, as an experiment, I tried a vegetarian diet for at least four months. In the first month, I felt good and light, but, starting with the second month, I did not feel well. I had to stop. I tested myself both before and after the experiment, and the results revealed that I had developed several nutritional deficiencies after four months of a vegetarian diet, especially a deficiency of vitamin B12. It makes so much sense because I grew up in a fishing village in the southern part of the Philippines. My childhood daily diet consisted of fish and vegetables. Today, I must eat a lot of green, leafy vegetables daily. Otherwise, I will be constipated.

Coming to America thirty years ago did not change my gut's metabolism and the function of my immune system. I have to be very careful not to overeat American food based on animal protein. I am more likely to get Type 2 diabetes from a diet of too much processed food and from a higher meat intake than I was used to while growing up. Another factor is the size of my liver and my pancreas. I have much smaller organs than those in the average body of northern European origin.

A 2005 study conducted by J. R. Speakman, PhD, DSc, at the Aberdeen Centre for Energy Regulation and Obesity (ACERO), School of Biological Sciences, University of Aberdeen, Aberdeen, Scotland, UK, linked the complexity of connection of the mitochondria's metabolism rate of free-radical generation between body size, metabolism, and lifespan. My body parts are a lot smaller in size, so I don't need that much food anyway. So, I also must watch my serving size. My eyes are usually bigger than my stomach, so having a smaller plate helps me pace my eating habits. There were no buffet restaurants when I was growing up in the Philippines in the 1970s.

 Pain is a friendly messenger. Self-healing is holistic and relies on you to provide the healthy raw materials and the right environment for healing.

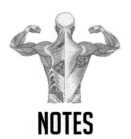

NOTES

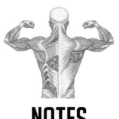

NOTES

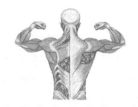

C H A P T E R 3
THE CAUSES OF DEGENERATIVE CHRONIC DISEASES

"As to diseases, make a habit of two things—
to help, or at least, to do no harm."
—Hippocrates

y professional medical journey of over thirty years has led me into an objective examination of the oversights and the limits of the Western model of health and healing. I am not alone in this position, though my perspective is far from conventional. Early on, I realized that the repertoire of remedies from the mainstream medical teachings and the thousands of scientific journals were massively inadequate. Indeed, the Western model's advances in therapeutic approaches and technological devices are very effective for acute and emergency trauma care. Unfortunately, the limitations and the failures of a single biochemical and surgical model have plagued the twenty-first century.

What has been missing in mainstream medicine is biophysics and epigenetics principles. Once I realized this, I began a journey in pursuit of effective restorative healing strategies that work to help patients with troubling degenerative diseases. I focused primarily on epigenetics. Diligently pouring over literature and available evidence led me to a form of practice that was unconventional but rooted in biomedical knowledge and science. I turned to therapies that worked. With an enthusiastic drive, I dove into the study of the ancient art of various medical systems, like the 3,000-year-old traditional Chinese medicine (TCM). It teaches a logical but straightforward biomechanism concept as the cause of degenerative disease. Understanding the biomechanics of conditions is the key to addressing the disease process head-on for healing.

CAUSES OF DEGENERATIVE DISEASES

In this section, I will briefly describe the rich medical system and concepts of healing in TCM. It started in China and spread worldwide. It is continuously practiced in most Asian countries and has been for almost twenty-three centuries. This ancient art is the practice of medicine that focuses on the prevention or healing of diseases by maintaining or restoring the balance of the two complementary forces, *yin* (passive) and *yang* (active). Good health in the TCM paradigm happens when harmony exists between these two forces. Illness, on the other hand, results from a breakdown in the equilibrium of *yin* and *yang*.[72]

The fundamental tenet of TCM is biophysics and applied epigenetics. It is a comprehensive practice of electrical-energy medicine, nutritional medicine, and biochemical or herbal medicine. Its practical components are acupuncture, herbs, lifestyle changes, emotions, and foods for healing.

A persistent blockage of or the absence of bioelectrical and biochemical energy may cause your body to be diseased. In the

TCM healing paradigm, there are two major biomechanisms for the causes of degenerative diseases:

1. Congestion and stagnation
2. Depletion and deficiency

Congestion and Stagnation
Congestion and stagnation are based on the premise that your body is full of freeways of plumbing and an extensive electrical network. If you were to lay out all the arteries, capillaries, and veins in one adult, end-to-end, they would stretch about 60,000 miles or 100,000 kilometers. These freeways of tubing and electrical wiring are connected and travel all over the body. Any epigenetic factor that blocks or slows the travel process down, thus the congestion and stagnation, will effectively cause degenerative disease to develop. For example, consistent massive harmful food intake and poor lifestyle choices will eventually block arterial and venous blood flow. These types of conditions respond well to cleansing and detoxification.

Congestion and stagnation are known to cause most degenerative diseases in the organs (such as the liver), in tissues, in circulation, in lymph, and in cells. The liver is a natural multitasker. It conducts more than 3,000 functions in the body. It plays a significant role in metabolism, helps build proteins, breaks down hormones, clears toxins from the bloodstream, and much, much more. A congested or stagnant liver will not put you in immediate danger. Still, it will produce significant symptoms—in this case, digestive problems—that can lower your quality of life and indicate that you are headed for trouble down the road. Changes in lifestyle—such as eating healthy foods, getting regular exercise, drinking plenty of water, and taking time to relax with good sleep—are often enough to bring the liver back into functional balance.[73] For example, weight gain is a symptom of congestion and stagnation, not a disease. It is a sign that something is off balance and not working.

The pathology of stagnation and congestion comes more likely from overeating, with poor bowel elimination, from overworking, and from weak stress-coping mechanisms. The best and fastest way to heal is for one to use cleansing and detoxification. These will let the rest of the internal organs repair and regenerate new body parts. This method is universally recognized as strengthening digestion. Detoxification helps the liver and other internal organs to process incoming nutrients and to filter impurities from circulation more efficiently.

Classic examples of congestion and stagnation are Type 2 diabetes, heart disease, or even cancer, based on the TCM paradigm. These diseases, especially at the early stages, can be resolved more quickly and efficiently with detoxification and cleansing.[74] Think about it: taking more medications when you have a disease of congestion and stagnation will cause your liver and your internal organs to be sicker and more congested! Why is it that modern medicine's first line of intervention with diabetes is typically medications instead of detoxification and cleansing?

Dr. Jason Fung, MD, a Canadian nephrologist, is a world-renowned author and medical clinician on intermittent fasting and a low carb diet, especially for treating people with Type 2 diabetes. In his book *The Diabetes Code*, he has successfully helped to cure and to reverse thousands of Type 2 diabetic patients with intermittent fasting as part of his medical intervention. For some of his dialysis patients, he even helped them wean off daily dialysis by following his dietary regimen.

Besides, a 2004 study by Mark P. Mattson, PhD, a professor of Neuroscience at Johns Hopkins University and the former chief of the Laboratory of Neurosciences, National Institute on Aging Intramural Research Program (along with his colleagues), suggests that intermittent fasting (IF), reduced meal frequency, and caloric restriction (CR) extend lifespan and increase resistance to age-related diseases in rodents and monkeys. These dietary protocols also improved the health of overweight humans.[75] We will discuss detoxification and fasting in Book Three.

Depletion and Deficiency
The second cause of most degenerative diseases is depletion and deficiency. Depletion and deficiency are physiological states in which there is a lack of one or more nutrients or not enough of one or more nutrients in the system for it to function optimally. This issue needs a different approach from the one used in the processes of congestion and stagnation. Nowadays, you can find out your exact deficiency of nutrients by performing nutritional testing, mitochondrial blood testing, or by physical exam. Once the deficient nutrients are identified, they can be replenished adequately. These nutrients are considered essential simply because your body does not manufacture them, like essential fatty acids or vitamin C.

It is essential to know that humans cannot manufacture vitamin C, but most animals, like cows and goats, do produce them efficiently.[76] Micronutrients must come from your daily nutrition of vegetables, fruits, and meats that are rich in essential vitamins and minerals. Otherwise, your body cannot correct itself back to health. This primary nutritional deficiency needs to be stabilized first up to a therapeutic level, and only then can fasting and cleansing can be beneficial.

Depletion and deficiency could also come from the lack of macronutrients, such as fats, proteins, and plant-based good carbohydrates, as well as from the lack of micronutrients, such as enzymes, minerals, and vitamins. You need continuous replacement of these essential macronutrients and micronutrients. As you perform your activities of daily living, your body undergoes a constant process of use and repair. All these activities require a continuous supply of the correct raw materials. Your body may allow or tolerate junk food or unhealthy substances that look like food, but it takes more energy and more work for the body to digest them. Not to mention that these bad foods assault and break down your gut and other internal organs faster than eating healthy. In addition, junk foods do not replenish essential macronutrients and micronutrients and do not prepare the body for growth; nor do they maintain health.

A classic example of severe vitamin C deficiency is *scurvy*. It is a life-threatening condition suffered by people who do not have access to fruits or vegetables for long periods. Vitamin C must be optimized to a therapeutic level to correct scurvy.

The human body is a solar-powered machine. You need to be outside; your skin needs the sun at least a few hours a day. Solar power is the primary source of your vitamin D3. Every cell of your body needs a constant supply of vitamin D3 to achieve optimal health. A deficiency or an absence of vitamin D3 will run havoc in your immune system. Without it, your body will become weak, fatigued, and more vulnerable to getting sick. The best remedy is to get a healthy dose of sunshine outside. More on this topic in Book Three.

Other examples of depletion and deficiency are osteoporosis, osteopenia, and osteoarthritis. These conditions are not healthy at any age. In my clinic, I have seen osteoarthritis in a patient as young as six years of age. Poor diet is the main culprit here. Contrary to common knowledge, osteoporosis and osteopenia are not due to a deficiency of calcium. Most people consume enough calcium in their diets. Calcium is a fat soluble nutrient.[77] Osteoporosis and osteopenia are more likely due to a lack of calcium cofactors. (This topic will be discussed more in the Calcium section in Book Three). The culprits are likely a fat-free diet deficient in vitamin D3 and essential fatty acids, poor sleeping habits, deficient essential minerals, and dehydration.[78]

PRIMARY DEGENERATIVE DISEASES

I call the following the *mother* or the *primary* degenerative diseases. Most clinical diagnoses will come from these five primary diseases. Some will have at least one or a combination of two or more problems in a person's disease process. It makes it easier to address the cause and to come up with a proper solution.

1. *Leaky-gut Syndrome*

Leaky-gut syndrome is a condition in which the intact walls of the gut, including the intestines, develop tiny holes, admitting substances into the bloodstream that would typically be excluded. Symptoms of the syndrome include bloating, gas, cramps, food sensitivities, and aches and pains. Conventional physicians do not generally recognize leaky-gut syndrome, but the evidence has been accumulating that it is a real condition that affects the lining of the intestines. Leaky-gut syndrome, also called "increased intestinal permeability," is the result of damage to the intestinal lining, making it less able to protect the internal environment, as well as less able to filter needed nutrients and other biological substances. Consequently, some bacteria and their toxins, fungi, parasites, fats, waste, and partially digested proteins may leak out from our intestines and into our bloodstream. This triggers an autoimmune reaction. Our body will begin to attack itself because of the presence of foreign particles in the blood.

It can eventually lead to gut problems, such as abdominal bloating, excessive gas and cramps, fatigue, food sensitivities, joint pain, skin rashes, and autoimmunity. Causes of this syndrome may be poor diet, chronic inflammation, food sensitivity, damage to the gut from taking large amounts of nonsteroidal anti-inflammatory drugs (NSAIDS) and cytotoxic drugs, radiation, taking certain antibiotics, excessive alcohol consumption, toxin exposure, infections, and compromised immunity. Leaky-gut syndrome can also be caused by another gastrointestinal disease or by poor liver function, resulting in inflammatory toxins being excreted into the intestines.

2. *Liver Congestion*

Your liver is the biggest organ in your gut, and it can perform more than 3,000 functions in your body. It can regenerate itself every six-to-eight weeks. It is working hard during the day and cleans itself at night. It makes all your red blood cells and washes all food you eat. It is the main helper for all your gut organs, like your pancreas, stomach, small and large intestines, and colon.

When your liver functions poorly or becomes congested, you are going to see a myriad of problems in your body: conditions like fatty liver disease (either from alcoholic drinks or nonalcoholic drinks), insulin resistance in type 2 diabetes, gall stones, obesity, and other metabolic syndromes.

For example, in nonalcoholic fatty liver disease (NAFLD), your liver is significantly congested. It means that your liver cells are storing too much fat. Fatty tissue builds up in your liver, whether you drink little or no alcohol. It is an umbrella term for a range of liver conditions affecting people who have poor eating habits, like high sugar and too much protein. It tends to develop in people who are overweight, obese, have diabetes, high cholesterol, or high triglycerides. There appears to be a connection between the disease and insulin resistance. When you eat, your liver helps blood glucose to enter your muscles. However, when your liver is sick, it will resist the insulin from going to your muscles—your body develops insulin resistance. It means that your cells do not respond to insulin the way they should. As a result, too much fat ends up in the liver. It will cause havoc and harm in all the over 3,000 liver functions—such as producing bile, which helps break down fats and remove waste from the body, producing immune factors to fight infections, metabolizing medication, and removing toxins, and many more. So, the best way to reverse NAFD is to heal your liver first by unclogging it through fasting. More about fasting in Book Three.

3. *Chronic Dehydration*

Every cell of your body is approximately 70 to 75 percent water. All biological functions need water for them to happen. Your kidneys need mild saline water to do their job in filtering toxins out of your body. Any other kind of beverage is extra work for your kidneys. What is fantastic about our bodies is that they are very forgiving. They can compensate for a short duration of dehydration. However, prolonged, unintended dehydration will cause significant clinical problems, like migraines, headaches, back and neck pain, arthritis, joint aches, and high blood pressure. When chronic dehydration becomes severe, it can lead to a significant health crisis, such as fibromyalgia, lupus, rheumatoid arthritis, and even cancer.[79] Recovery time for dehydration depends on the underlying cause and may also depend on how long you have been dehydrated. More on water in Book Three.

4. *Nutrient Deficiency*

Your body needs all the right macronutrients and micronutrients to survive. It also requires all the vitamins, enzymes, and minerals to function optimally. Any significant depletion of any of the necessary nutrients will cause clinical conditions. For example, low vitamin C will give you problems fighting infections, bleeding into joints, and severe joint pains. However, a severe deficiency of vitamin C will result in scurvy. Symptoms include fatigue, depression, and connective tissue defects (for example, gingivitis, petechiae, rash, internal bleeding, impaired wound healing). Once you figure out what the nutrient deficiency is, the nutrient needs to be replenished before your body can be healthy again.

When you suffer from symptoms of nutrient deficiency, you are not deficient in medications. You need to shape up and start addressing the problem by eating healthy. In the worst cases, please consult your holistic health practitioner. More on nutrients in Book Three.

The word "toxin" comes from the Latin word "toxicum," meaning "poison." A toxin is any substance that can poison or cause harm to an organism, an organ, a tissue, or a cell.

Toxins, in this discussion of applied epigenetics, are very significant. The toxin's role is to create a negative environment or even an external assault on our physiology. It can turn on the gene expression of disease. A toxin can come in many different forms, either natural or human-made. There are generally four types of toxic substances: chemical, biological, physical, and those from radiation. Today, there are six specific sources of toxins—namely, ingested or food-based poisons, external poisons, environmental poisons, emotional poisons, intellectual poisons, and spiritual poisons.

Toxicity is the degree of damage to an organism from one or more toxins. Toxicity harms the whole body, as well as impacts the basic unit of an organism, like a cell or an organ, such as the liver. Physiologically, the adverse effects of toxicity can block a function or can deplete nutrients that will eventually lead to a disease process.

In addition, the word "toxicity" can be used to describe toxic effects on more substantial and more complex groups, such as the family unit or society at large. Toxicity can also cause emotional, intellectual, social, and spiritual damage. Sometimes, the word is more or less synonymous with poisoning in everyday usage.

Toxicity can be measured by its effects on the organism, the organ, the tissue, or the cell. However, individuals typically have different levels of response to the same dose of a toxin because the effect of the toxin on an individual is dose-dependent and based on their bio-individuality. The toxic dose is dependent on the amount, the duration, and the rate of frequency of toxins used. Even water can be toxic when taken in too high a dose.

In contrast, a highly toxic substance, like cyanide, ingested at a minimally effective dose, can be extremely poisonous, causing immediate damage, like sudden death, to an organism. In addition, a slow, constant, and prolonged exposure of minute doses of cyanide can show obvious damage only after a specific period. Maybe most of you have heard of natural and human-made toxins, but I would like to highlight their adverse role in the cell's epigenetics mechanism. More on detoxification in Book Three.

I have mentioned toxicity as one of the causes of primary degenerative diseases. In the next chapter, I will discuss, in detail, all forms of toxins that you find in food, cosmetics, personal hygiene products, as well as emotional, spiritual, and intellectual toxins.

 Most degenerative diseases have two basic mechanisms: congestion and depletion.

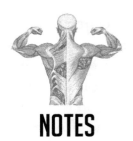

NOTES

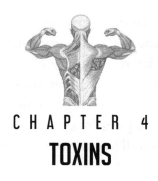

CHAPTER 4
TOXINS

"Illnesses do not come upon us unexpected. They are developed from small daily sins against Nature. When enough sins have accumulated, illnesses will suddenly appear."
—Hippocrates

Every year, environmental pollutants worldwide have caused more than 13 million deaths.[79] In addition, approximately 24 percent of diseases are caused by environmental exposures that might be mitigated through preventive measures.[79] Rapidly growing evidence has linked environmental pollutants with epigenetics variations, including changes in DNA methylation, in histone modifications, and in microRNAs.[80]

According to an environmental chemical exposure screening survey conducted by the United States Center for Disease Control and Prevention, 148 different environmental chemicals were found in the blood and urine in the U.S. population.[81] Growing evidence suggests that environmental pollutants may cause diseases via changes in gene expression regulated by epigenetics mechanisms.[82]

The good news is that ongoing scientific studies are evaluating the effects of environmental exposures on the epigenome. Such studies are trying to determine if the effects can be mitigated by positive changes in lifestyles or can be worsened by the interaction with other risk factors. Future epigenomic research may provide information for developing preventive strategies, including exposure reduction, as well as pharmacological, dietary, or lifestyle interventions.[83]

Toxins versus Nutrients

It is essential to know the difference between these two words: "toxins" ("poisons") and "nutrients." The food industry is guilty of massaging the truth about healthy nutrition. For the past fifty to sixty years, there has been so much misinformation about proper nutrition. The food industry has been efficiently manufacturing food-like products. Also, the power of food marketing continues to spread misinformation about the real definition of food. Wrong information about food kills more people than all cancers and other diseases combined. The misleading advertising is dangerous and has led to more harm.

We need to go back to basics. Let us begin by defining "food." Food is any substance consumed to provide nutritional support for our body's survival. It is usually of plant or of animal origin which contains essential nutrients, such as carbohydrates, fats, proteins, vitamins, and minerals. Food is ingested by an organism and assimilated by the organism's cells to provide energy, to maintain life, or to stimulate growth.

Now let us define a "nutrient." A nutrient is any substance that, when ingested, nourishes our body with nutritional enzymes. Nutrients replenish the body with the necessary enzymes that keep the body healthy. Food enzymes come from organic, locally grown fresh vegetables and fresh fruits, as well as from meats from animals raised in pastures.

Once the food is digested, it has a positive or negative impact on your body. Food can contain a nutrient or a toxin or both. Nutritious foods contain more useful molecules that nourish and support your body. On the other hand, toxic foods contain particles that could cause harm to your body. They can deplete or block nutrients from being absorbed. Toxins can be natural-based or human-made, and these toxins can be put into the food. Toxins can weaken the body's defenses by taking away essential nutrients. Toxins can also be either biological, like pathogenic bacteria in food, or chemical, like most prescription drugs. Sugary foods can cause nutrient depletion by taking away magnesium.

A toxin can also dehydrate you, such as caffeine. Your coffee or any caffeinated drink can dehydrate you because of caffeine's diuretic effect on the body, which dries up your cells. Your kidneys are using more water just to separate water from caffeine. Caffeine's neurostimulant effect may wake up brain cells, but it also dries them up overall. Just keep in mind that drinking coffee is not hydration. Hydration should remain your priority first thing in the morning since your body is 75 percent water. It needs that much water to function optimally. See more on the water in Book Three.

Eventually, toxins can build up. They can clog up the body's systems, especially your liver. Toxins can slow down your liver's physiological functions, and can even cause degenerative diseases.

It is critical to keep in mind the difference between nutrients and toxins when you make food choices for you and your loved ones. There are only two kinds of food: real whole food and manufactured, or processed, food. Real whole food is food in its original and complete state. It is produced from mother nature, without being manufactured or processed. Being able to differentiate between real whole food and manufactured, or processed, food (also called "junk food") when navigating the grocery stores and reading labels is very critical. The easiest way to shop in the grocery store is to check the foods displayed throughout the periphery, especially the fresh produce section. Just be aware, it is by design that 80 percent of the packaged foods are conveniently placed in the middle section. For seven years, I have taught Epigenetics 101 class. One of the vital lessons in my class is understanding food labels and familiarizing with real and fake ingredients used in the food manufacturing.

Our body's activities use up a lot of energy. The body needs to be consistently replenished with the right nutrients. It also needs to be hydrated with the correct fluid, primarily water! Eating and hydrating will surely give you energy. The quality of energy is dependent on the quality of the right food choices: real, whole, or manufactured.

Taste is *not* a good criterion by which you can differentiate between nutrients and toxins. The food industry has mastered taste science to perfection, but it does not prioritize maintaining the maximum nutritional integrity of your food. The food industry is a master at making food taste conveniently good so that you may forget to question whether it is healthy for you or not. The standard American diet contains manufactured artificial flavors geared only toward sweet or salty. Real healthy food, with high nutrients, has a variety of tastes. It can be bitter, a little spicy, or a bit salty. According to TCM, your lymphatic system, one of your defense systems, functions better with bitter-tasting vegetables and good healthy fats.

Let us take a look at a typical American breakfast, which consists, in part, of a bowl of cereal. For almost sixty years, cereal in its many forms has been heavily marketed as a healthy, fiber-filled breakfast. Even the American Heart Association has stamped its official seal of approval on the cereal box. One bowl of cereal, such as cornflakes, contains approximately sixty grams of added sugar, not to mention the milk sugar, called lactose, in it. By the way, one regular breakfast bowl is equivalent to two serving sizes of cereal. Yes, cereal indeed contains dietary fiber, but the fiber is heavily coated with sugar and artificial food coloring to make it taste and look good. The toxins overshadow the nutrients so that the cereal is empty and bereft of the fresh, essential, whole-food nutrients that are necessary for growth and maintaining life. Most cereals are the worst breakfast anybody could eat. Boxed cereal is a food-like substance. In fact, the cereal box is healthier than its contents, since the box has more fiber from the paper pulp from which it was made.

There are two significant kinds of toxins. First are natural toxins, which are natural substances. They cover a large variety of molecules generated by fungi, algae, plants, or bacteria, with harmful effects on humans or other vertebrates, even at minimal doses. The second is human-made toxins. These toxins are chemicals or biological substances intentionally added during the manufacturing of everyday products, like plastics, cosmetics, personal products, and medications.

FOOD TOXINS

Food toxins are poisonous, human-made chemicals or processes that are intentionally put in our food during manufacturing. They are added in the processing of foods to improve taste, shelf life, and marketability, for the sake of the almighty profits, while compromising food's nutritional value. We will begin with a list of the top eighteen modern-day, food-based toxins you *do not* want in your diet.

1. *GMO – Genetically Modified Organism*
GMO is the acronym for the term genetically modified organism; its genome has been engineered in the laboratory to favor the expression of desired physiological traits or the production of desired biological products. A genetically modified organism (GMO) is a heavily engineered agricultural crop that was genetically designed initially for resistance to pathogens and herbicides. It is widely marketed as having better nutrient profiles and drought tolerance.

GMO opponents have popularly nicknamed "Franken foods." The modification process sometimes involves inserting a gene from an animal into a plant, like a goat gene or a virus gene into an apple or spinach. Precision crossbreeding in GMOs between plants and animals is very unnatural. In GMO technology, scientists in a laboratory can move one trait, maybe from a plant or from an animal, with precision, to produce some new quality or some unique characteristic onto a plant product.[84]

For the past fifteen years or more, GMO crops, through genetic technologies, have become a part of our everyday life. They are used in twenty-nine countries worldwide—one-tenth of the world's farmland. Most GMO crops are grown in America, and they account for one of our most significant exports to the world. Genetic modification has practical applications in agriculture, in food production, in medicine, in research, and in environmental management, although it is still highly controversial in its impact on our digestive and immune systems. Scientific research is increasingly showing evidence that a constant diet of GMO foods wreaks havoc on gut flora, which can eventually lead to leaky-gut syndrome.[85]

The groundbreaking book *Silent Spring* by Rachel Carson indicates that genetically engineered agricultural pesticides have a massive negative impact on our gut health.[86] They directly or indirectly affect the systemic physiological problems that we see in children's diseases today. There is an epidemic-scale health crisis, especially regarding our children's health. The pediatric population, especially, should not be fed GMO products since children's gut flora are still very immature and weak.

Agricultural scientists have used radiation and chemicals to induce gene mutations in edible crops, in attempts to achieve desired characteristics. For example, a GMO apple has an added anti-browning gene to keep it from oxidizing or decaying; a GMO pink pineapple is genetically enriched with the antioxidant lycopene. The five most common GMO crops are corn, canola, soy, cotton, and sugar beets. Corn syrup, oil, sugar, flavoring agents, thickeners, and other ingredients are used as additives in all kinds of packaged foods. In an average grocery store, roughly 75 percent of processed foods contain GMOs. Most GMO wheat grains are high in lectins because they have been modified to fight off bugs, and they are also heavily treated with toxic pesticides.

In 1994, a Canadian study was performed on glyphosate residue in the seed and straw of wheat. It showed that the physiological maturity of the crop, the rainfall wash-off, and the application rate of pesticides appeared to play essential roles in determining the magnitude of glyphosate residues.[87] This means that GMO wheat seed may contain a variable concentration of the super pesticide called glyphosate. The level of concentration will depend on the agricultural farming technique, how much pesticide was used, the farm environment, and precisely the amount of seed moisture in which it was grown. This simply means that, within the crop season, the concentration of the pesticide present in the wheat seed depends on the amount of the pesticides you apply, the number of times you use it, and the dryness of the seed crop. Sadly, the consumer does not know how much pesticide they are consuming at a given moment because it is not rigorously tested. There is also no requirement to declare the pesticide content on the stuff you buy in the grocery store. To add insult to injury, the cumulative amount of pesticides in all the food you eat daily is unknown.

I am seeing, in clinics across the country, a chronically sick population, especially children. They are all suffering as unknowing participants in several decades of experimentation with the daily dose of genetically modified manufactured foods. Sadly, no long-term GMO studies have ever been done on humans. Only animal studies have been done, and results are not good.

A 2007 study published in the journal *Archives of Environmental Contamination and Technology* showed that rats fed with Monsanto's MON863 corn for more than ninety days began to show signs of toxicity in the liver and the kidneys. In 2001, Russian biologist Alexey V. Surov released the results of a study testing the effect of Monsanto's genetically modified soy on hamsters. After monitoring three generations over two years, Surov learned that third-generation hamsters not only lost the ability to reproduce but began growing hair inside their mouths.

An Australian study published in November 2008 showed that the more genetically modified (GM) corn was fed to mice, they had fewer and smaller babies.[88] In Haryana, India, a team of investigating veterinarians reported that buffalo consuming GM cottonseed suffer from infertility, as well as from frequent abortions, premature deliveries, and prolapsed uteruses. Many adult and young buffalos have also died mysteriously.

As Alexey V. Surov, a Russian biologist, says, *"We have no right to use GMOs until we understand the possible adverse effects, not only to ourselves but to future generations as well. We need fully detailed studies to clarify this. Any type of contamination has to be tested before we consume it, and GMO is just one of them."*

In December 2013, more than 300 scientists, physicians, social scientists, academics, and specialists in legal aspects and risk assessment of GMO crops and foods signed a landmark petition. They demanded strong scientific evidence about the long-term safety of GMO crops and foods for human health, animal health, and environmental health. Such evidence must be obtained in a manner that is honest, ethical, rigorous, independent, transparent, and sufficiently diversified to compensate for bias.[88] After two years, a follow-up study, performed in 2015, resulted in no scientific consensus on GMO safety.[89] The authors of this study claimed, "Governmental bodies' endorsements of GMO safety are exaggerated or inaccurate."

2. *Sugar: the Antinutrient*

There is no getting around it: we Americans have a sweet tooth. The average sugar consumption of most Americans is about twenty-two teaspoons per day, which amounts to seventy-seven pounds of sugar per year. Sugar is very toxic to the liver, which is why it is called hepatotoxic. Sugar, especially fructose, is metabolized in the liver as harmful fat.[90] It feeds the growth of yeast, candida, harmful bacteria, and, most of all, the rapid growth of cancer. Harmful bacteria create toxins called exotoxins, which damage healthy cells and can eat a hole in your intestinal wall. Thus, too much sugar, as well as a constant consumption of sugar, will weaken the gut lining. The human gut was simply not made to hold excessive amounts of sugar. Sure, you're probably not sucking on sugar cubes throughout the day, but you are probably downing more than your fair share of sugary cereals, snacks, sodas, ice cream—and the list goes on and on.

Sugar is known as the antinutrient also because it is a compound that is very toxic to the body. However, sugars, such as glucose, are an essential structural component of living cells and a source of energy in many organisms. The term "simple sugars" denotes "monosaccharides," each of which contains a sugar consisting of one molecule. The term "table sugar" or "granulated sugar" refers to sucrose, which is a disaccharide. It has two single sugars: glucose and fructose. It is ideal to limit both types of sugar combined intake to fifteen grams per day.

Sadly, modern agricultural techniques have changed the fruits we eat. In 2018, the Melbourne zoo stopped feeding its animals with fruits. "The issue is the cultivated fruits have been genetically modified to be much higher in sugar content than their natural, ancestral fruits," Michael Lynch, the zoo's head veterinarian, told the *Sydney Morning Herald*. In addition, Dr. Senaka Ranadheera, a food scientist at the University of Melbourne, said there were reports of some fruits, such as plums, almost doubling in soluble sugar content in the past twenty years. Based on these developments, it is ideal to minimize one's fruit intake because fresh fruits have been engineered to be more significant in size and to have increased sugar content up to 50 percent more than their counterparts in the 1970s.[91]

Clinical studies have supported the conclusion that sugar glycation thickens the blood and causes a metabolic assault on the body's immune system and aging.[92] I strongly recommend watching the YouTube video by a pediatric endocrinologist, Dr. Robert Lustig, MD, entitled, *Sugar—The Bitter Truth*. He passionately explains his clinical findings, based on his forty-year clinical experience, that sugar is the number one cause of heart disease and diabetes.

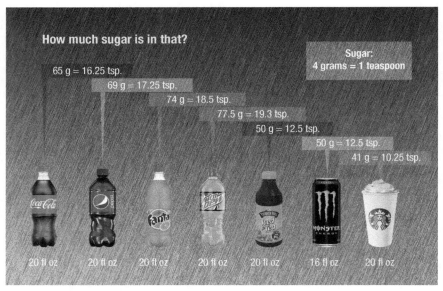

FIGURE 5. Beverage Sugar Content Comparison

According to William Dufty's book, *Sugar Blues*, eating five grams of sugar suppresses your immune system for four hours. If you are fighting a cold or the flu while eating any sugary foods, it will take you longer to recover because you have handcuffed your immune system.

We could also apply this argument to cancer. Cancer cells, for example, can use about 200 times more glucose than healthy cells, which often results in different sugars displayed on their surfaces than healthy cells.[93] Most cancer cells need a massive amount of sugar to fuel their growth, according to a noted cancer researcher director of the Meyer Cancer Center at Weill Cornell Medicine in New York, Dr. Lewis Cantley, PhD.[94] Other cancer experts say sugar itself can drive cancer. Dr. Peiying Yang, PhD, a cancer researcher and associate professor at MD Anderson Cancer Center in Houston, concurred with Cantley on the strong correlation between high insulin levels all the time and a higher risk of cancer. It is not only that cancer loves to feed on sugar, but it also suppresses your immune system. So, when you give a cancer patient sugary protein drinks, you are feeding the cancer, not the patient.

3. *Artificial Sweeteners*
Artificial sweeteners are fake sugars. We already know that real sugar is very toxic. Fake sugars are 1,000 percent more toxic. Avoid all counterfeit sugar products! Sucralose (Splenda), aspartame (NutraSweet), saccharin, and neotame are all fake sugar products, promoted as "sugar-free" products.

How sweet is fake sugar? The relative potency of sugar compared with artificial sweeteners shows how much sweeter the latter are: sugar 1×, cyclamate 45×, aspartame 180×, saccharin 300×, sucralose 600×, neotame 13,000×. These products are not sugars—they are nonnutritive food! They may taste sweet to trick your tongue and brain, but they do not trick your stomach at all. Your gut knows they are junk! These nutrient-empty sweeteners will hurt every cell of your body.

Americans are slaves to their tongues' sweet taste buds. Last year alone, the food industry introduced 2,225 reduced-sugar and "sugar-free" foods. They were consumed by at least 250 million people worldwide. The use of artificial sweeteners is highly controversial. Some claim that artificial sweeteners are entirely harmless, but new studies suggest that they may have adverse effects on your metabolism.[95] The long-term health effects are still unclear, and health authorities like the FDA do consider all artificial sweeteners to be safe. I disagree. There is no debating that these artificial sweeteners are bad for you. They are unnatural and very toxic to your gut. They are another of those human-made fake foods. They are no better and could be worse than real sugar.

Let us look at the history of these artificial sweeteners.

Aspartame

The FDA approved aspartame in 1974. But it has been plagued with controversy since 1980. Regardless, it has gained popularity for public consumption in the United States, the United Kingdom, and the European Union. Aspartame is the primary sweetener found in brand names like Equal® and NutraSweet®.

Scientist James M. Schlatter accidentally discovered aspartame in 1965. As Schlatter was researching an anti-ulcer drug, he licked his finger to get a better grip, and the sweetness he tasted was aspartame. Aspartame is a human-made artificial sweetener made by combining two amino acid proteins: aspartic acid with phenylalanine. Once digested, it breaks down into methanol and formaldehyde in your small intestines. Methanol is a form of alcohol, while formaldehyde is the same compound for embalming dead bodies. It doesn't sound very healthy and appealing, once you know what it is, does it? If your gut could talk to you, it would ask, "Why?"

Aspartame is about 200 times sweeter than regular table sugar. The idea was that less aspartame was needed to achieve the same sweetness as regular table sugar, with lower calorie intake, as well, thus helping with weight loss.

Over the years, several claims have been made against aspartame, from causing blood-related cancers (leukemia and lymphoma) to headaches, dizziness, depression, weight gain, ADHD, digestive problems, and mood changes.[94] I am not surprised by these claims. Your body's digestive system is brilliant, but it is designed to digest real food, not fake food. You cannot trick your body and get away with it.

Sucralose

Sucralose is another artificial human-made sweetener. Splenda® is composed of 95 percent sucralose and 5 percent maltodextrin. Maltodextrin is a highly processed compound made from corn, rice, potato starch, or wheat. Sucralose was discovered in 1976 when a scientist at Kings College in London misheard instructions about testing a chlorinated substance. He tasted his mistake and realized that it was highly sweet.

Sucralose is 400 to 700 times sweeter than table sugar, without the bitter aftertaste many other artificial sweeteners have. The idea, again, is to achieve the same delicious taste with fewer calories. Sucralose has zero calories. And maltodextrin has three calories per teaspoon.

As expected, adverse effects of sucralose consumption are being reported. Insulin and blood sugar have been elevated by as much as 20 percent; gut bacteria have been reduced by 80 percent after twelve weeks of sucralose use; and, when heated at high temperatures with glycerol (the backbones of fat molecules), sucralose will produce chloropropanols, which may raise the risk of cancers.

Saccharin Sodium

Saccharin sodium is the oldest artificial sweetener and has been used for over 100 years; it was made in a laboratory in 1865. It is commonly known today as Sweet'n Low®, Sweet Twin®, and NutraSweet®. Saccharin sodium became popular in the 1960s and 1970s as a sugar replacement. It may come as a surprise to many who remember the controversy in the 1970s when studies linked the sweetener to bladder cancer. Countries around the world, including the United States and Canada, decided to ban the sweetener as a food additive.[96] In 2000, the FDA declassified saccharin sodium, declaring it safe again for human consumption.

Saccharin sodium is 300 to 400 times sweeter than regular table sugar, but it is known for its metallic aftertaste. It is used in carbonated diet drinks, low-calorie candies, jams, jellies, and cookies, as well as in many vitamins and medicines.

In 2010, the Environmental Protection Agency removed saccharin sodium from its list of hazardous materials. However, ingesting saccharin sodium may still cause some side effects, such as the increased risk of cancer, diabetes, allergic reaction, and weight gain.

Neotame

Neotame is the new kid on the block among the nonnutritive toxic sweeteners and is produced under the trade name Newtame. It is aspartame on steroids.

It is 7,000 to 13,000 times sweeter than table sugar. Sadly, it is allowed in organic foods. It may be an even-more potent and more dangerous neurotoxin, immunotoxin, and excitotoxin than aspartame. Neotame makers and supporters claim that its toxicity is negligible because it is consumed only a little at a time. Ironically, such a claim is like saying it is okay to ingest a poison slowly.

If you have ever wondered what the adverse effects of neotame might be, I suggest that you refer to the list of detrimental effects of aspartame and multiply them by an exponential power as being hazardous to your cells. In short, it is super bad for you!

4. *Gluten*

Gluten is a group of proteins (gliadin and glutenin) that are found in the starchy part of the endosperm of various cereal grains.

Gluten is the glue from grains that is potentially damaging to your intestinal lining, causing leaky-gut syndrome. Gluten is a protein complex that accounts for 75 to 85 percent of the total protein in bread wheat. It gives elasticity to dough. It helps bread to rise and to keep its shape, and it often gives the final product a chewy texture. It acts as a powerful glue that binds food together.

Recently, there have been increasing numbers of adverse reactions to gluten, especially in America. "Gluten-related disorders" is the umbrella term for all diseases triggered by gluten, which include celiac disease (CD), nonceliac gluten sensitivity (NCGS), wheat allergy, gluten ataxia, and dermatitis herpetiformis (DH).[97] Currently, their incidence is increasing in most geographic areas of the world. There are many explanations for the rise of these disorders: (1) the growing Westernization of diets; (2)the increased use of wheat-based foods in the Mediterranean diet;[98] (3) the progressive replacement of rice by wheat in many countries in Asia, the Middle East, and North Africa;[99] (4) the development in recent years of new types of wheat grain with more cytotoxic gluten peptides; and finally, (5) the reduction of dough-fermentation time, owing to a higher content of gluten in wheat and resulting in less time for baking bread and bakery products.[100]

People can also experience adverse effects from wheat because of a wheat allergy. As with most allergies, a wheat allergy causes the immune system to respond abnormally to a component of wheat that the immune system treats as a threatening foreign substance. This immune response is often temporary and does not cause lasting harm to body tissues.

When people have weak stomach linings, they will have a hard time digesting gluten. Undigested proteins are toxic. Once an undigested gluten protein escapes into the bloodstream, people will develop gluten intolerance symptoms. If such symptoms are left uncorrected, over time, gluten may eventually interrupt brain proteins and the metabolism of the gut, or it may inflame the gut and cause conditions like colitis, irritable bowel syndrome (IBS), leaky-gut syndrome, or celiac disease.

Patients eating gluten from any source may complain of mild-to-severe symptoms. It is an excellent idea for you to have a blood test if you suspect gluten intolerance or worse. You may benefit from a gluten-free diet to heal your gut lining. Please consult a good holistic health practitioner to help you with your gut and gluten issues. A good reading suggestion is Dr. David Perlmutter's book, *Grain Brain: The Surprising Truth about Wheat, Carbs, and Sugar—Your Brain's Silent Killers.*

5. *Lectins*

Lectins are antinutrient proteins that bind tightly with carbohydrates. The bond is so powerful that our natural digestive enzymes are unable to break it apart. It is hard on our intestinal walls to break these proteins down, so they could cause a tear in the walls over time. Lectins are found in some beans, fruits, vegetables, nuts, seeds, grains, and cereals. Cooking and digesting lectins destroy some but not all of them. As a result, some beans, such as kidney beans or pinto beans, are inedible when raw and ought to soak in water for at least twenty-four hours before they are cooked. Most grains and legumes are indigestible until they are prepared adequately; they need to be soaked for twenty-four hours before they are cooked.

Lectins are the plant's biochemical defense mechanisms. A lectin is the plant's strategy to protect itself from being devoured by pests, including humans. It is Mother Nature's biochemical warfare to prevent the plant's extinction. It is also the plant's protection against pathogens, like parasites. It also helps in the plant's protein synthesis and delivery in animals. It is an antinutrient that consists of relatively sticky molecules, which make it useful in binding with its sought-after sugars, but it is undesirable for our digestion. Lectins have strong binding powers that can lead them to attach to the intestinal lining and to wreak havoc.

Over the ages, traditional cultures have progressed in their techniques for food preparation. Humans were able to figure out how to predigest or to neutralize lectins through proven, traditional ways of preparing food, such as fermenting, sprouting, and soaking. However, in our modern, instant-food practices, we tend to skip these ancient, proven practices, thereby wreaking havoc on our digestive system.

6. *Phytates*

Phytates are antinutrients similar to lectins, but they can be beneficial phytonutrients. Phytates bind with minerals, such as iron, calcium, and zinc, and reduce or block their bioavailability in your gut, possibly leading to deficiencies, especially if your diet is high in fiber and whole-grain foods.

Phytates have eight different names; the most common are "phytic acid," "inositol hex phosphate," and "IP-6." Phytate, or phytic acid, is the principal storage form of phosphorus in many plant tissues, especially bran and seeds. Phytates store the phosphorus needed to support germination and growth. Plants have phytate enzymes, but humans do not. The human gut bacteria are not healthy enough to digest phytates.

The problem with unsprouted grains, beans, and nuts, including wheat, rice, and spelt, is that they may contain large amounts of nutrient blockers such as phytates and lectins. Poorly prepared soybeans, pinto beans, kidney beans, and navy beans, as well as peanuts, have a high content of phytates and lectins.[101] They have double the amount of phytates found in peas, lentils, chickpeas, white beans, walnuts, and mung beans. Unlike grains, which have a large concentration of phytates in the bran, phytates are concentrated in the seeds. It is essential to know that potatoes also contain phytates.

Traditional ways of preparing food, such as soaking, fermenting, and sprouting, are the most effective ways to neutralize the effects of phytates. You need to soak rice, beans, and raw nuts for at least four hours and up to twenty-four hours, with a teaspoon of aluminum-free baking soda, before cooking them. This technique can reduce phytates by 50 percent, according to the Weston A. Price Foundation. When beans are sprouted, the total phytate level goes down by as much as 75 percent. Sprouting retains nutritional value, but the longer you soak and cook food, the more essential vitamins and minerals you will lose, together with the phytates.

7. *Food Coloring*

Food involves more than just taste; the appearance of your food is just as important to entirely appreciate what you eat. The processes of our digestive system start when we see the food before we even taste it. There is a logical link between color and taste. Much of what we eat would not look appetizing if it were not in color. Food coloring is cosmetics for your food to entice your eyes. Without coloring, hot dogs would be gray.

Naturally, oranges are orange, and we expect orange-colored drinks to be orange flavored. Red drinks should taste like cherries, and purple drinks should taste like grapes. If a portion of food is gray, it could be moldy and should not be eaten, unless you are eating blue cheese—which gets its distinct flavor from mold!

There are two kinds of food coloring: natural food coloring and artificial or synthetic food coloring. For centuries, natural dyes have been used to color food to make it more appealing.

The most common natural dyes are carotenoids, chlorophyll, anthocyanin, and turmeric.

1. Carotenoids have a deep red, yellow, or orange color. A carotenoid is a fat-soluble, bright orange pigment found in sweet potatoes, pumpkins, and carrots. It is also used for yellow coloring in dairy products, like cheese or margarine.

2. Chlorophyll is the natural green pigment found in all green plants. During photosynthesis, this green pigment absorbs the sunlight and converts it into energy, to make carbohydrates from carbon dioxide and water.
3. Anthocyanin is an organic compound that is the best natural source for deep purple and blue. It is the central molecule of the vibrant colors of grapes, blueberries, and cranberries. It is a water-soluble dye, which is perfect for water-based food products, such as blue corn chips, brightly colored soft drinks, and jelly.
4. Turmeric is another ancient plant-based food dye. It is indigenous in India and is used as the spice curcumin. When turmeric is found in mustard, it will turn a deep yellow. Turmeric is also an excellent acid or base indicator. If you add a basic substance to mustard, the mustard will turn red.
5. Carminic acid is a deep-red dye. It is an animal-based coloring that comes from a bug called a "cochineal." The Aztecs have been using these insects to dye fabrics in a deep-red color for centuries. If you crush up to 70,000 of these bugs, you can extract a pound of deep-red dye. It is found in various food and cosmetic products that require a red color, like your vibrant, red lipstick.

Artificial food colorings were initially derived from coal tar, which comes from coal. Today, most synthetic food dyes are derived from petroleum or crude oil. One stain that does not have a petroleum base is Blue No. 2, or indigotin, which is a synthetic version of the plant-based indigo dye; indigotin is used to color blue jeans.

It is important to note that some of the natural dyes may cause severe allergic reactions in some people, like saffron and annatto, which is used for yellow food coloring. There is some scientific evidence that children who consume food coloring will show gut intolerance symptoms.[102]

Substantial evidence has shown that most artificial food colorings from coal tar or petroleum products, like yellow, red, and blue food color, will burden our kidneys and liver.[103] It is hard to purge them out of the body. They tend to stay in the brain or in other, weak organs.

8. *Soy Products*

Unfermented soy products such as tofu, soy milk, soy infant formula, and soy meat have become popular and more accessible since the turn of the century. A meatless product comes from texturized vegetable protein. Because of extensive advertising, many consumers believe that these products are healthy meat alternatives for protein in their diets. According to Kaayla T. Daniel, PhD, CCN, in her book, *The Whole Soy Story: The Dark Side of America's Favorite Health Food,* unfermented soy causes thyroid dysfunction, cognitive decline, reproductive disorders, infertility, and even cancer and heart disease.

Soy is the raw material for the best glue commercially produced and used in industrial applications. Soy-based glue is the preferred industrial glue for permanently securing the glass window on high-rise commercial buildings. Soy-based glue can withstand intense environmental assaults, like strong wind shear, extreme heat, and extreme cold, day in and day out.

Soy foods such as those mentioned above contain antinutritional factors such as saponins, soya toxin, phytates, protease inhibitors, oxalates, goitrogens, and estrogens. Some of these factors interfere with the enzymes you need to digest protein. Soy has an isoflavones-a type of phytoestrogen, which is a plant compound resembling human estrogen. These compounds mimic and sometimes block the hormone estrogen and have adverse effects on various human tissues. Soy phytoestrogens are known to disrupt endocrine function, may cause infertility, and may promote endometrial cancer in women.[104]

According to a 2007 study conducted by C. Duffy and his colleagues, there is very little human data on the role of phytoestrogens in preventing breast cancer recurrence. Still, the few studies conducted do not support a protective role.[105] It is also suggested that soy's phytoestrogen genistein may interfere with the inhibitive effects of tamoxifen on breast cancer cell growth.

In contrast, fermented soy products, like other fermented vegetables, are beneficial to your digestive system. The long fermentation process reduces the phytate and antinutrient levels of soybeans, which can act as toxins in your body and cause gastric distress and low absorption of nutrients. The friendly bacteria or probiotics found in fermented soy help nourish the gut and digestive flora, boosting digestion and the absorption of nutrients. Because most of the immune system resides in your stomach, these beneficial fermented soy products aid immune function, too. One example of such products is tempeh, a fermented soybean cake with a firm texture and a nutty, mushroom-like flavor. Miso is a fermented soybean paste with a salty, buttery texture (commonly used in miso soup). Natto is fermented soybean with a sticky texture and a firm, cheese-like flavor. Soy sauce is traditionally made by fermenting soybeans, salt, and enzymes.

9. *Pesticides*

Pesticides are toxic by design—they are biocides, designed to kill, to reduce, or to repel insects, weeds, rodents, fungi, or other organisms that can threaten public health and the economy.[106] Pesticides pose serious risks to human health and safety. Because of their widespread use, people in every part of our food system— producers, workers, and consumers—can be exposed to potentially harmful levels of pesticides.

Research has shown that pesticides and other agricultural chemicals are neurotoxins and can mess up your brain.[107] The Environmental Protection Agency (EPA) considers 60 percent of herbicides, 90 percent of fungicides, and 30 percent of insecticides to be carcinogenic. All these toxins are allowed on conventional farms. Any number of them can end up on your plate when you purchase conventionally grown fruits and vegetables.

An FDA sampling of nearly 6,000 foods revealed that fruits and vegetables are most frequently contaminated with pesticide residues. Notably, 82 percent of domestic fruits and 62 percent of local plants had such residues. Eating non-organic, genetically engineered foods (the prime candidates for Roundup spraying) is associated with higher glyphosate levels in your body. A study of close to 4,500 people in the United States found that those who often or always ate organic produce had about 65 percent lower levels of pesticide residues compared to those who ate the least amount of organic produce.[108] So, choosing organic foods as much as possible is a crucial way to lower your exposure to pesticides.

If you must choose which products to purchase, choose organic, grass-fed animal foods and organic produce. The Environmental Working Group's (EWG) released the Dirty Dozen list, which ranks the twelve items most heavily contaminated with pesticides. As of 2017, these include strawberries, spinach, nectarines, apples, peaches, pears, cherries, grapes, celery, tomatoes, sweet bell peppers, and potatoes. For the non-organic produce you consume, washing with a solution of baking soda may help to remove some of the pesticides on the surface of the fruit or the vegetable. However, it will not remove chemical residues that have penetrated beyond the peel.[109] A 2013 study found that phenoxy herbicides, such as 2,4-D, had some of the highest abilities to transfer through the orange peel. The investigators determined that, in the skin of five oranges and five mandarins purchased from stores in Vietnam, the 2,4-D content in oranges (79 to 104 µg/kg) was significantly higher than that in mandarins (1.66 to 2.82 µg/kg).[110]

10. *Hormones and Steroids*

In this section, I will address hormones and steroids together, since they are commonly used in conjunction with each other. They both create the same adverse effects on humans. Hormones and steroids are given to livestock to improve profits from dairy and meat, like beef, chicken, fish, and pork. Recently, the pervasive use of hormones and steroids in our food supply, particularly in animal husbandry, has become more controversial because of increasing public awareness and education about their harmful effects on the human body.

The most widely used hormone is the recombinant bovine growth hormone for increasing milk production for dairy cows, while estrogen, testosterone, and progesterone are consistently fed to beef cattle to promote growth. According to the U.S. Food and Drug Administration (FDA) and a joint committee of the Food and Agricultural Organization and the World Health Organization (FAO/WHO), the amount of these hormones and steroids that make it into food products is negligible and is not harmful.[111] They adamantly endorsed that it is fit enough for human consumption, but is it?

The insulin-like growth factor-1 (IGF-1) plays an essential role in milk production, bone growth, and cell division, both in humans and in cattle. It is safe to assume that humans can absorb extra IGF-1 from milk, thus increasing its level in human blood. According to the pediatrician Dr. Michael Woods, MD, FAAP, *"Higher levels of IGF-1 in the blood may be associated with an increased risk of some cancers, but no evidence has proven a link. The same connection has been made to estrogen levels and risk of breast or ovarian cancer, although again, no evidence is present at this time."*

It is a given that high levels of hormones and steroids can cause problems in the human body. The big question is: Do the accumulated hormones and steroids from meat and dairy that we eat harm our body? As of today, there are no long-term studies that have shown evidence of a reliable connection between the dangers of or the safety of consuming hormones and steroids in animal meat on humans. However, because of consumer demand, some buyers and store chains are beginning to promote and to sell hormone-free and steroid-free meat products. Some countries have banned hormones and steroids, specifically to prevent harming animals, but not for helping humans.

I have a problem with this slow-dose poisoning in our food supply. I think we have grossly underestimated the adverse health outcomes on the lifetime exposure to hormones and steroids daily in our epigenome health. It can gravely affect our population, from infants in utero to people of all ages and to the next generations to come.

Until more extensive, long-term research is done, it is best to err on the side of caution. According to the scientists and the medical authorities that do advise caution, prepubescent children are at the highest risk. Pregnant women may also want to use educated discretion.

To keep hormone-treated and steroid-treated products off your and your family members' plates, you need to buy meat that originates only from animals organically pasture-raised and 100 percent grass-fed and finished. The animals cannot be given steroids or hormones. In addition, you should buy meat products from your local organic farm or from a biodynamic, small-scale farm. They have, by far, the best meat products for your health. In short, the traditional and local, small-scale family farming needs to come back. They are our best hope and the backbone for our optimal health.

11. *Antibiotics*
An intensive animal feeding operation (AFO) is one in which over 1,000 animal units are confined for over forty-five days a year. One animal unit is equivalent to 1,000 pounds of live animal weight.[112] Let us do the math: 1,000 animal units × 1,000

pounds of live animal weight = 1,000 cows, 700 cows used for dairy purposes, 2,500 pigs weighing more than fifty-five pounds (twenty five kilograms), 125,000 chickens, or 82,000 egg-laying hens or pullets.[113] An AFO is not the same family farming we have idealized. This is farming on steroids, literally and figuratively!

To prevent the animals from being sick while being farmed in their congested and filthy environment, they are consistently given antibiotics and fed with highly processed corn or soy-based feeds. Not to mention when cows are given a consistent dose of rBGH, they are prone to udder infections or nipple and breast infections (mastitis) because the high use of antibiotics can create resistance to certain bacteria.

Residues of pesticides in the industrialized corn- and soy-based feeds and veterinary drugs, such as antibiotics, are in these animals' meat. The residues will eventually enter our food system when producers bring animals to slaughter that still have these toxins in their system. Beef, pork, and chicken can all be affected.

Farmers use hormones and antibiotics to increase growth or to cause weight gain, to treat infection, or to keep the animals healthy. Constant exposure to contaminated meat by humans will eventually weaken their livers and immune systems and can lead to resistance to those antibiotics in the food. When you build up resistance to certain antibiotics, antibiotics may no longer work, just when you need them the most. Shop wisely for organic or other meat that is labeled as being sourced from animals that have not been treated with antibiotics or hormones.

12. *Pasteurized Milk*

Cow's milk contains the essential amino acid A1 casein—which serves as a building block for new muscles. It is the most abundant protein in cow's milk. It is relatively insoluble. It is a macromolecule that is hard to digest in your gut without the proper enzymes. The amino acid A2 casein, from sheep, goat, and buffalo, is a much smaller molecule, compared to the cow's amino acid A1 casein. It is the reason why goat's milk is more easily digestible than cow's milk.

Pasteurization is a process that uses acid or mild heat, usually to less than 100 °C (212 °F), to eliminate pathogens and extend the shelf life of milk. Pasteurization is done to minimize the total bacterial count of milk, resulting in reduced chances of spoilage. Through this process, the casein peptides and micelle structures become disturbed or denatured. The enzymes are a critical factor in raw milk. When you cook or pasteurize the milk, you kill all the enzymes. The live enzymes and the good bacteria that digest lactose are destroyed, thus destroying the nutritional and enzymatic value of milk. Daily ingestion of the antibiotic tetracycline present in pasteurized milk causes a public health concern because it can increase the resistance of microorganisms to antibiotics.[114]

If you're suffering from insulin resistance and if you're overweight, you may want to limit your milk consumption, as milk has significant amounts of lactose and galactose—simple sugars that may worsen insulin resistance and make it more challenging to lose weight. In fact, you may stay away from drinking reduced-fat or skim milk. According to Dr. William Winter, DVM, cofounder of the American Holistic Veterinary Medical Association (AHVMA), full-fat raw milk actually tends to modulate the impact of the milk sugar, and people who stick to a low-fat diet tend to be more overweight. He considers reduced-fat or skim milk to be junk food.

"The Nine Reasons to Stop Drinking Any Kind of Pasteurized Milk," taken [115] from the article written by Natasha Longo[116] are:

1. Pasteurization masks low-quality milk. Dairies rely on heat treatments to mask their inferior sanitary conditions. It can have pus, manure, and debris. Consumer Reports found 44 percent of 125 pasteurized milk samples contained as many as 2,200 organisms per cubic centimeter, like fecal bacteria, coliforms.

2. Pasteurization destroys nutrients like calcium, vitamin C, and damages water-soluble B vitamins. In high heat called a Maillard chemical heat reaction, the proteins and sugars turn brown, discoloring the milk.

3. Pasteurization destroys enzymes, vitamins, proteins, and antibodies as well as beneficial hormones, making it dead milk. Live milk enzymes help digest lactose. Both enzymes and milk proteins help absorb vitamins. Once these protective enzymes are dead, pasteurized milk is more susceptible to spoilage. Vitamin C loss in pasteurization usually exceeds 50 percent; loss of other water-soluble vitamins can run as high as 80 percent. The Wulzen or anti-stiffness factor is totally destroyed.

4. Pasteurized milk can trigger mast cells to release histamines, causing asthma. The histamines flooding, in turn, lead to inflammation, mucus production, and bronchial spasms. Dairy is one of the most inflammatory foods in our modern diet, second only to gluten.[117] Pasteurization warps and distorts the fragile proteins, which causes allergies.

    Unpasteurized milk heals and prevents asthma by neutralizing mast cells and maybe reducing inflammation if you are not allergic to it.[115] Rebuild immunity by keeping the good bacteria to colonize the gut and become immune protective and improve the digestive ecosystem.

5. Pasteurized milk can cause diarrhea, cramps, bloating, gas and gastrointestinal bleeding, iron-deficiency anemia, skin rashes, atherosclerosis, and acne. It can also cause recurrent ear infections in children. It also causes insulin-dependent diabetes, rheumatoid arthritis, infertility, and leukemia.[118] The fact that pasteurized milk puts an unnecessary strain on the pancreas to produce digestive enzymes, may explain why milk consumption in civilized societies has been linked with diabetes.

The protein lactalbumin in milk is a critical factor in diabetes—a good reason for NOT giving cow's milk to infants. You may try rice-based baby formula milk or make your own homemade rice milk. Just be careful that it has essential nutrients that will be needed to grow a healthy baby. CAFO cows are fed with corn and soy, not grassfed in the pastures. Eighty-nine percent of America's dairy herds have the leukemia virus.[119] Cows diagnosed with John's Disease have diarrhea and heavy fecal shedding of bacteria.[120] These bacteria become cultured in milk. They are not destroyed by pasteurization.

6. Pasteurized milk harms bone density. The dairy industry has been hard at work for the last 50 years, convincing people that pasteurized dairy products such as milk or cheese increase bioavailable calcium levels. It is false. The pasteurization process only creates calcium carbonate, which has absolutely no way of entering the cells without a chelating agent. So, what the body does is pull the calcium from the bones and other tissues to buffer the calcium carbonate in the blood.

This process causes osteoporosis.[121] Pasteurized dairy contains too little magnesium needed at the proper ratio to absorb the calcium. Most would agree that a minimum amount of calcium to magnesium ratio is two to one and preferably one to one. So, milk, at a cal/mag ratio of ten to one, has a problem. You may drink 1200 mg of dairy calcium in milk, but you will be lucky to absorb a third of it into your system. Over 99 percent of the body's calcium is in the skeleton, where it provides structural stability. Pasteurized dairy forces lower calcium intake than average, and the skeleton is used as a reserve to meet the body's needs.

Long-term use of skeletal calcium to meet other physiological needs of the body leads to osteoporosis. Dairy is pushed on Americans from birth, yet Americans have one of the highest incidences of osteoporosis in the world. A 12-year broad study based on 77,761 women aged between 34 and 59 years of age in the Harvard Nurses' Health Study found that those who consumed the most calcium from dairy foods broke more bones than those who rarely drank milk.[122]

The test for pasteurization is called the negative alpha phosphatase test. When heated milk is at 165 degrees (higher for ultra-heat treated or UHT milk) and pasteurization is complete, the enzyme phosphatase is 100 percent destroyed. Guess what? It is the enzyme that is critical for the absorption of minerals, including calcium!

7. Pasteurization kills antibiotic effectiveness for all of us.

Pasteurization created a dairy farm system that relies heavily on antibiotics fed to heifers and dry cows at CAFO, mega-dairies that support massive milk production. The antibiotics now used in American hospitals for humans no longer work. Tens of thousands of Americans now die each year because of superbugs created by CAFO antibiotic abuse.[123] MRSA and VRA drug resistance are now a significant cause of death. There are fewer, and sometimes no antibiotics left to kill the bad bugs and save human lives. The FDA has conceded antibiotic use in farm animals must be phased out but refuses an outright ban or limit of the use of antibiotics in CAFO feed.[124] The FDA instead testifies in defense of antibiotic use by the CAFO industry.

8. Pasteurization fuels cancer. Of the almost 60 hormones, one is a powerful growth hormone called Insulin-like Growth Factor One (IGF-1). By a freak of nature, it is identical in cows and humans. Consider this hormone to be a fuel cell for any cancer. The medical world says IGF-1 is a critical factor in the rapid growth and proliferation of breast, prostate and colon cancers. We suspect that most likely, it can promote ALL cancers.

IGF-1 is a normal part of all milk, intending to help the newborn to proliferate! What makes 50 percent of obese American consumers think they need more growth? Consumers do not think anything about it because they do not have a clue about the problem nor do most of our doctors.

9. Pasteurization kills cows on green pastures. Seventy-five years ago, there were friendly cows in green fields all over America. Pasteurization has excellently paved the meadows and now forces the cows to be fed soy protein concentrates and forty pounds of grain per day, along with antibiotics and hormones. This CAFO dairy feeds increase milk production to numbers never seen before in the history of the earth. It is common for some CAFO dairy cows to produce twenty gallons of milk per day. The cows are placed into pens deep in manure with thousands of other cows. The stress of being milked up to four times per day and lying on artificial rubber beds shortens their lives to just forty months. A cow living on pasture will produce much less milk, four to five gallons per day, and comfortably live ten years or more in pure bliss and health.

13. *Farm-Raised Seafood*

Farm-raised seafood is unnaturally fed with corn or other grains, as well as with soy or other legumes. As a result of this economical, but unnatural, diet, levels of critical omega-3 fats may be reduced by about 50 percent in farmed salmon compared to wild salmon. The seafood tanks or pens of farm-raised seafood, much like the enclosures of crowded farm animals raised for slaughter, can become polluted and contaminated by seafood waste and uneaten food. This contamination, in turn, can lead to disease. Farm-raised seafood is often treated with pesticides and antibiotics to fight infection and parasites.

14. *Fluoride*

Studies have been done on the effects of fluoride on children in China, and the results suggest fluoride is as toxic to the human brain as lead or mercury.[125] Fluoride exists naturally in groundwater and is more prevalent in some areas of China. The studies showed that children in high-fluoride areas had significantly lower IQ scores than those in low-fluoride areas.

15. *Mercury*

Mercury is a toxic heavy metal, one that can cause harmful effects to your nervous, digestive, respiratory, and immune systems. The mercury used in dental amalgams (fillings) and thimerosal (a mercury-based preservative added to flu vaccine vials) have been linked to autism in children. Mothers with dental amalgams were more likely to have children with autism than mothers without them. Resin-based fillings are safer alternatives to dental amalgams. There are thimerosal-free flu vaccines available, as well, so that both hazards can be avoided.

For over 150 years, dental amalgams have been widely used for restorative tooth fillings, especially in posterior teeth, because of the amalgam's high mechanical strength, durability, ease of manipulation, and low cost. A dental amalgam is an alloy composed of approximately 50 percent elemental mercury and a mixture of other metals, such as silver, tin, copper, and sometimes palladium, indium, and zinc. This is how toxic your dental amalgams are. If one of your dental amalgam fillings were dropped in Lake Conroe, that lake would be declared contaminated with poisonous mercury materials. The Environmental Protection Agency (EPA) would swarm that place in a heartbeat. No swimming or any activity would be allowed.

Despite the known toxicity of dental amalgams, it is still legal for dentists to use them in your mouth. Every time you eat acidic food, the mercury-filled amalgam will release microscopic particles into your digestive system, compromising your immune system. Cancer patients with dental amalgams are advised to have them carefully removed by a certified biologic dentist to mitigate the toxin load and to boost their immune systems.

Recent cell phone studies have shown the effect of radiofrequency radiation from the Wi-Fi device or cell phones' microwave emissions.[126] According to Maryam Parnahad, and colleagues, a 2016 study concluded that radiofrequency radiation emitted from Wi-Fi devices significantly increased mercury release from amalgam restorations.[127] A cell phone interacts with any metal next to its location of use. For example, the 2016 study was able to detect the increase of radiofrequency radiation of your dental amalgam when the cell phone is placed next to the tooth for twenty minutes, like pressing the cell phone against your cheeks while talking.

16. *Chlorine*

Chlorine is a very close cousin to the iodine molecule in the chemical periodic table. Chlorine is a chemical bully to iodine, who is a friend of the thyroid. Your thyroid hormone uses iodine to activate T3 from T4. Without iodine, your thyroid function will slow down into low-active-thyroid levels or low-thyroid symptoms. Chlorine, which is used in your tap water, pool water, and in bleaching products, can weaken your thyroid. Most people take warm or hot, steamy showers that open pores and increase absorption.[128] When the chlorine touches your skin, while you are taking a bath or swimming in highly chlorinated tap water, it will be absorbed into your bloodstream in seconds![129]

The best remedy is to filter your tap water either by a whole-house-reverse-osmosis filter system or by a shower head chlorine filter that costs $30.00. Make sure to change the filters every three months, especially if your tap water is highly chlorinated. Always drink filtered water, never tap water!

According to the U.S. Council of Environmental Quality, "*The cancer risk to people who drink chlorinated water is 93 percent higher than those who do not.*"[130] A CDC report concludes that there is a probable link between chlorine and perfluorooctanoic acid (PFOA) in the water supply.[131] It causes high cholesterol, ulcerative colitis, thyroid disease, testicular and kidney cancers, as well as pregnancy-induced hypertension. PFOA in water supplies is a waste byproduct of the manufacturing process.

17. *Food Preservatives*

Food preservatives, such as Butylated hydroxyanisole (BHA) and Butylated hydroxytoluene (BHT), lengthen the shelf life of foods. They are linked to health problems, such as cancer, allergic reactions, and more. The International Agency for Research on Cancer classifies BHA as a possible human carcinogen.[132] Food preservatives can affect the neurological system of your brain, can alter behavior, and can cause cancer. The European Commission on Endocrine Disruption has also listed BHA as a Category 1 priority substance, based on evidence that it interferes with hormone function.[133] Tertiary butylhydroquinone (TBHQ) is a chemical preservative so deadly that ingesting just five grams can kill you.[134] The preservative sodium benzoate has been found to cause children to become more hyperactive and distractible. It is found in many soft drinks, fruit juices, and salad dressings. Sodium nitrite, a common additive to hot dogs, deli meats, and bacon, has been linked to higher rates of colorectal, stomach, and pancreatic cancers.

18. *Microwaved Food*

Avoid all microwaved food. Heating food can always result in some nutrient loss, but heating food by microwave can have a drastic effect on its nutritional value. The November 2003 issue of *The Journal of the Science of Food and Agriculture* found that broccoli zapped in the microwave with a little water lost up to 97 percent of the beneficial antioxidant molecules it contains.[135] By comparison, steamed broccoli lost 11 percent or fewer of its antioxidants. Another study on bread baked in the microwave showed a 70 to 75 percent decrease in the protein amino acid. Intermolecular and intramolecular cross-linking of gluten was formed in microwaved bread.[136]

Another study on microwaving breast milk found that it destroys the essential disease-fighting agents in breast milk that offer protection for your baby. This 1992 study found that microwaved breast milk lost lysozyme activity and antibodies and that it fostered the growth of more potentially pathogenic bacteria.[135] According to the author, microwaving has done more damage to the milk than other methods of heating.[137]

Microwaving is using ionizing radiation to cook your food. It heats the water molecules in food, which causes the particles to rotate rapidly in the microwave. The faster the water molecule rotates, the more molecular friction it creates. The friction produces heat that heats your food. Most of the food nutrients will be degraded because of water loss during the microwaving process. Microwaving your food can also dry it. In addition, cooking your food in the microwave can strip away its original nutrients, as well as killing its enzymes. For example, microwaved bread becomes very hard. When one of the bread sugar molecules reaches 212°F (100°C), it melts, which softens the bread. It is why bread can feel soft and fluffy when it first comes out of the microwave. But when it cools, that molecule recrystallizes and hardens, causing the bread to become chewy and hard.

Studies have also suggested that microwaving food could change its DNA. A 2009 study on the nonthermal levels of microwave exposure showed that microwaving food can produce single- and double-strand breaks in DNA in solution.[138] It is alarming to me. Nuking your food to heat it seems faster, but, realistically, you saved only a few minutes; indeed, you will lose a lot more! You will lose your food nutrients, and you are messing with your food's DNA. Yikes!

Furthermore, when plastic is heated, toxic chemicals, like BPA and phthalates, can leach out of the containers or the covers, contaminating your food with endocrine and hormone disruptors.

A paper published in 1990 reported the leakage of many toxic chemicals from the packaging of typical microwavable meals, including pizzas, chips, and popcorn.[139]

19. *Caffeine*

Caffeine acts as a central nervous system stimulant. According to the U.S. National Library of Medicine, high doses of caffeine can cause significant health issues, including rapid or irregular heartbeat, heightened blood pressure, shakiness, dizziness, anxiety, seizures, sleep problems, and unintended diuresis.[140] Caffeine will irritate the gut wall and dehydrate the body. Caffeine metabolism varies from person to person. Some people do not have enzymes to metabolize caffeine; they suffer from what is called "caffeine sensitivity." There is also what is called "a slow metabolizer," a person having a genetic makeup with a slower rate of caffeine processing. As a result of slow processing, caffeine may have longer-lasting stimulant effects.

Dr. Fereydoon Batmanghelidj, MD, in his book *Your Body's Cries for Water*, states that he used water as a treatment, mainly by necessity, when he was a political prisoner at Evin Prison, in Tehran, Iran, from November 1979 to May 1982. He was able to examine about 3,000 patients and to follow the medical fate of more than 600 fellow prisoners. For three years, he performed experiments using water and coffee, a known diuretic agent. He found that if you drink one cup of coffee, it takes your kidney three-to-four cups of water to separate water from caffeine. It seems that caffeine takes more water and more work for your kidney.

Caffeine dehydrates the body, especially the brain and the kidneys, and it weakens the bladder. It is a diuretic that produces more urine in the body. Caffeine also blocks the brain enzyme PDE (phosphodiesterase), which is essential to expanding memory. Caffeine can cause anxiety disorders in people who were otherwise free of mental health pathologies. Caffeine users are more likely to be depressed.

Studies have found that prolonged caffeine use makes you emotionally anxious. In other words, continued caffeine intake will increase your propensity to be emotionally concerned. In a 1997 study published in the *Journal of Psychopharmacology*, of the British Association of Psychopharmacology (BAP), the investigators found clinical evidence of caffeine-induced anxiety, lower tolerance to stress on continued use, and withdrawal anxiety in chronic caffeine-containing beverage users.[141]

ENVIRONMENTAL TOXINS

Environmental toxins are cancer-causing chemicals, bioelectrical magnetic irradiation, and endocrine disruptors. These toxins are both human-made and naturally occurring, and they can harm our health by disrupting sensitive biological systems. Environmental toxins can be found in our everyday lives: in the air we breathe, in the water we drink, and in the electromagnetic fields created by Wi-Fi in our homes.

Give some thought to the air quality where you live and how you can maximize your exposure to air that has not been contaminated by smog and pollution. Air pollution can cause a variety of illnesses in humans, including asthma, lung cancer, heart disease, and even reproductive and developmental disorders.[142] It can also compromise the immune system by overworking the respiratory system and the body's natural defenses.[143]

Environmental toxins include naturally occurring compounds such as lead, mercury, radon, formaldehyde, benzene, and cadmium. They also contain human-made chemicals, like drugs, medications, parabens, phthalates, sulfates, BPA, artificial dyes, and pesticides. Here are the six most prevalent environmental toxins.

1. *Medications*

Medications, or drugs, are physiologically tough on the gut, intestines, liver, and kidneys. Medicines are right for you only if they address pressing acute symptoms. They are ideal when they are used for a relatively short period, maybe three to six months, at the most, to achieve a short-term goal and to minimize their adverse effects. The long-term remedy ought to be directed toward changes in lifestyle, exercise, and diet. Hence, this is where applied epigenetics is most effective. All medications are trying to mimic the function of raw healthy food, water, sleep, or exercise, but they can never come close to their incredible healing capabilities.

For example, pain medications can cause severe constipation. They will stop your intestinal muscles from contracting (peristalsis), preventing any movement of your bowels. Usually, after one week of pain medication, you will need a potent stool softener, or you will suffer the wrath of a constipated bowel.

Most medications are not designed to be taken for more than a month or certainly not years. After prolonged use of drugs, they will act as slow poisons. Always take probiotics and fermented foods after a course of medicines, especially after antibiotics regimen. It will help to remove any remaining residual medications and will reset your gut health.

2. *Parabens*

Personal-care products, such as sunblock, moisturizers, cosmetics, and hair products, can all be sources of toxins that have the most potential to be absorbed by your body. They get into your bloodstream directly through your skin pores. Just imagine your daily use of lotion spread across a large amount of skin, which may be there for some time, maximizing its potential to be absorbed. Many of these types of products contain parabens, cheap and effective preservatives that prevent the growth of bacteria and other microorganisms, thus prolonging shelf life.

Parabens are in all kinds of hygiene products, like shampoo, toothpaste, cosmetics, or creams, that you use daily. And they are sometimes used as food additives. You need to avoid them! Parabens contain xenoestrogens (XEs), chemicals that mimic estrogen in the body. It is this fake estrogen hormone that has lethal effect on the body causing several severe and pernicious health issues. According to Edwin Routledge, PhD, a molecular endocrinologist and an aquatic ecotoxicologist, *"Though we may only be exposed to trace amounts of these hormone imitators daily, they likely accumulate in the body and can build up to more dangerous levels over time, while also exerting a constant low level effect."*[144] Slow toxic poisoning is like the frog being slow-cooked in a pot: so subtle that you willingly pay money to put it in your body daily.

3. *Phthalates*

Phthalates are chemical compounds that are found in plastics— ingredients that give plastics their elasticity and that also change the texture and the quality of skin-care products. They are found in a wide variety of consumer products, including toys, cosmetics, pharmaceuticals, as well as in building and construction materials. Check the ingredient label for words ending in *phthalate*, as well as in *butyl ester* and *plasticizer*. Just like parabens, phthalates are considered testosterone and estrogen disruptors. Phthalates are found everywhere in our environment: in the chemicals we ingest, in the chemicals we put on our skin, and in the chemicals we inhale.[145] They are antiandrogenic, which simply means that they make testosterone worthless or even work against it, hence the term "anti-testosterone." They can cause reproductive problems, especially in males.[146]

In 2003, male reproductive problems were found in animal studies, while the animals were still in the womb.[145] Exposure to phthalates has been referred to as *phthalate syndrome*. It included decreased anogenital distance (AGD), infertility, reduced sperm count, cryptorchidism (undescended testes), hypospadias (malformation of the penis, in which the urethra does not open at the tip of the organ), and other reproductive-tract abnormalities.[147]

In addition, phthalates cross the placenta in humans,[148] as well as in animal amniotic fluid.[149] They also have been indicated as causing fat-related health risks[150] because phthalates tend to attach to the fatty tissues of the body.

4. *Sulfates*

Sulfates, including sodium lauryl sulfate (SLS), sodium laureth sulfate (SLES), ammonium lauryl sulfate, and sodium myreth sulfate, generally act as detergents or foaming agents and are found in cleansers and shampoos. The FDA regards SLS as safe as a food additive. Tests showed that SLS can penetrate the eyes.[151] SLS changes the amounts of some proteins in eye-tissue cells of all ages. It also affects such organs as your brain, your heart, and your liver.[152] These tests showed long-term retention in those tissues, mainly when used in soaps and shampoos. It is especially important in infants, where considerable growth is occurring and because a much higher uptake occurs in the tissue of younger eyes.

SLS forms nitrates. When SLS is present in shampoos and cleansers containing nitrogen-based ingredients, it can form carcinogenic nitrates that can enter the bloodstream in large numbers.[153] SLS can cause eye irritations, skin rashes, hair loss, scalp scurf like dandruff, and allergic reactions. SLS also produces nitrosamines, potent carcinogens that cause the body to absorb nitrates at higher levels than nitrate-contaminated foods, like hot dogs or luncheon meat.

5. *BPA*

BPA stands for Bisphenol-A. BPA is an industrial chemical used to make some plastic bottles and other cosmetic containers. Some research has shown that BPA can leak from the container into the contents of the bottle. Exposure to BPA is a concern because of the possible health effects of BPA on the brain and the prostate gland of fetuses, infants, and children.[154] It can also affect children's growth and development and behavior. Additional research suggests a possible link between BPA and increased blood pressure.[155]

Based on brain poisoning by BPA, anxious parents can take preventive measures to lessen infants' exposure to BPA: breastfeeding regularly, avoiding the use of dishwashers, and avoiding heating or boiling polycarbonate bottles. Instead, use BPA-free plastic bottles made of polyethylene, polypropylene, or glass.[156] Children and adults should be encouraged to use glass, paper, cloth, stainless steel, or ceramic packaging, as well as bottles for food and beverages.

6. *Preservatives and Dyes*

Preservatives and dyes in your cosmetics, personal products, clothing, furniture, and other household items can also harbor toxins. One such example is imidazolydinil urea, a preservative, which the EPA lists as toxic and which releases formaldehyde. Triethanolamine (TEA) is another chemical that can irritate the eyes, the skin, and the respiratory system, with long-term contact causing asthma and allergies.

A good rule of thumb for your hygiene products, including soap, deodorant, shampoo, and cosmetics, is to choose products that have five or fewer ingredients. That is a good sign that the manufacturer is providing a healthy product that will get the job done without introducing toxic preservatives, dyes, and other chemicals. Please read and carefully research the ingredients. If you do not know an ingredient or cannot pronounce it, then do not eat it, do not put on your skin, and do not even try to breathe it!

7. *Electromagnetic Radiation*

According to the EPA website, you can limit your exposure to electromagnetic radiation (EMR) by limiting your time spent near power lines and by increasing the distance between your body and the power source. Phones and computers emit EMR continuously. Electric fields are electric charges, and magnetic fields are the flow of electrical current through wires or electrical devices. Because of this, low-frequency EMR is found near electrical sources. As current moves through a power line, it creates a magnetic field called an electromagnetic field (EMF). The strength of the EMF is proportional to the amount of electrical current passing through the power line. It decreases as you move farther away. Because of this electrical property, your exposure to an electromagnetic field you would receive from a power line, from smartphones, from computers, and from wireless routers decreases with distance.

So, for starters, avoid living near strong sources of electromagnetic radiation. These include smart meters, radio stations, electrical generators, power lines, and electrified train tracks. Inside the house, keep electronic devices away from your body, such as cell phones, tablets, and computers. Keeping them out of the bedrooms helps to limit sleep disruptions from the EMF. Generally, unplug any appliances or devices that you are not using, including your Wi-Fi overnight. *Earthing* also can protect us from some of these human-made electromagnetic fields, especially from low-frequency EMFs.

Now, by this point, you may feel like giving up all the toxins you're surrounded with! How is it possible to make a difference in the way you live if there are environmental toxins everywhere? The truth is that you have more control than you think. Be intentional about your daily decisions, and research what you put into your body.

EMOTIONAL TOXINS

One toxin that is just as important as any other involves whom you spend time with and what information you allow into your mind and your heart.

Other internal toxins that we have more control over than we might think are emotional toxins. By this, I mean negative emotions or ways of thinking, stress and toxic relationships. It is best to master the art of positive thinking and to avoid cycles of self-hatred or self-doubt. The more positive attitude and positive internal conversations you have, the better able you will be to handle stressful situations, and the less likely you will be prone to illness.

Take some time to reflect on the situations or things in your life that stress you out. Can you find the root causes of the stress? Is the root cause a person, a job, or a busy lifestyle?

Consider the people you encounter in your life, how they make you feel, and what they bring to your relationships. Are they honest, caring, sharing, and communicative? Or do they think only of themselves, blame you or others whenever anything goes wrong, and take advantage of other people? If you know people who fall into the latter category, you are likely in a toxic relationship. Consider what kind of influence you have over these people. Eliminating toxic behavior and surrounding yourself with supportive, loving people will go far in creating and maintaining a healthier you.

MENTAL AND INTELLECTUAL TOXINS

Pornography is a twenty-first century epidemic. It has become the new addiction in this digital modern world we live in nowadays. According to U.S. researchers Jensen and Dines, pornography is *"sex divorced from intimacy, loving affection, and human connection. All women are constantly available for sex and have insatiable sexual appetites. And all women are sexually satisfied by whatever the men in the film do."*[157] Pornography is an unnatural act, not designed for our health.

All mammals, for the most part, have the same reward center in the brain. The reward center drives us to pursue things that improve our chances of survival and the survival of our genes, including food, sex, love, and novelty.[158] To steer us toward something that will help us, the reward center uses two different pleasure systems, one that excites and another that satisfies. The first system motivates us to go after things; it is dopamine that fuels it. The second system makes us feel satisfied and happy after accomplishing something. Endorphins run it.

Pornography activates both the reward center's pleasure systems, but the wanting system is stronger than the satisfying system. Pornography hyperactivates our wanting system, pumping out dopamine in response to each new image. As a result, the user can get caught in a loop of wanting, using, pumping out a bunch of dopamine in response to new images found while using, and then wanting even more.

A survey of 28,000 young Italian men found that they were suffering from sexual anorexia and were thus unable to get erections because of internet porn use that started in their mid-teens.[159] It also found that many Italian males started an excessive consumption of porn sites as early as the age of fourteen and that, after daily use in their early- to mid-twenties, they became enamored of "even the most violent images," according to Dr. Carlo Foresta, MD, a professor at the University of Padova and the head of the Italian Society of Andrology and Sexual Medicine (SIAMS).[157]

The side effects of pornography include pornography-induced erectile dysfunction (ED) and the shrinkage of the frontal lobe or the gray matter in the brain.[160] According to Dr. Nora Volkow, MD, the director of the National Institute on Drug Abuse, using illegal drugs like meth and cocaine (which overstimulate the brain's reward center with dopamine) can cause the brain's frontal lobes to shrink. Scientists have also found this type of shrinkage in the brains of people who have problems with natural rewards, such as overeating.[161]

Porn-addicted men are more likely to suffer from erectile dysfunction, according to lead researcher Dr. Matthew Christman, MD, a staff urologist with the Naval Medical Center in San Diego.[162] They are less likely to be satisfied with sexual intercourse, according to survey findings presented at the American Urological Association's 2017 annual meeting in Boston.

Pornography negatively contributes to mental and emotional health because of reduced dopamine.[163] It is associated with lower risk-taking in life and with increased anxiety, as well as with an increased likelihood for angry overreaction and with an inability to focus, as well as with a lack of motivation. More obviously, it gives the users a tendency for internet addiction, and it results in difficulty in maintaining healthy relationships, with a 2.5 times higher incidence of depression, anxiety, stress, and social problems.[164]

People who are addicted to pornography display intimacy problems, exhibiting decreased sexual and relationship satisfaction and changed sexual tastes.[165] They correlate with a lowered quality of life and poorer health, accompanied by an increased risk of harming themselves.[166] Some porn addicts also experience problems in memory, concentration, and impulse control.[167]

Doomsday and fear-mongering media sources are toxic to our mental and emotional health, as well. Constant exposure to doomsday news and fear-mongering media will set your body in a downward spiral into a sympathetic overload. Physiologically, your body will be in a survival mode, even without any real physical danger. When we watch the news on our televisions, phones, or computer screens, our brains have not completely evolved to recognize that the news stories are usually not present dangers.

Social media use is a relatively recent phenomenon. Sadly, it has become the primary form of communication for young people in the US and globally. Undoubtedly, using social media can be beneficial, including a source of social support and knowledge acquisition. However, a mounting body of evidence suggests associations with poor mental health among young people.[168]

Also, the recent rise of digital addiction in the social media networking craze adds insult to injury. Online social networking has caused profound changes in the way people communicate and interact. What is scary about social media's digital addiction is that it is so pervasive. It has the hallmark of the same mental rewiring of a cocaine- or gambling-addicted brain. Every time you get an alert on your social media, your mind feels an immediate high.

Your brain is pumping out a dopamine high, which is an exact mechanism as a cocaine-addicted brain. Several studies have indicated that the prolonged use of social networking sites (SNS), such as Facebook, Twitter, Snapshots, and other social media outlets, may be related to signs and symptoms of depression.[169]

Many studies have found a link between time spent using social media and mental health issues, such as depression and anxiety.[168] What is so alarming is that it afflicts all ages. Parents of infants and young children are recklessly using smartphones and portable electronic devices as digital pacifiers and digital playmates. It is a fact that adolescence is a period of vulnerability for developing depression,[170] and young people with mental health problems are at higher risk of poor mental health throughout their lives.[171] Social media will add a massive layer of developmental challenges for young school children, teenagers, and young adults. They are primed for depressive symptoms due to online harassment, sleep deprivation, self-esteem attacks, and distorted body image as victims and/or perpetrators. Digital addiction rewires their brain, resulting in stunting the emotional and social intelligence development necessary for lasting and real human interactions. This lack of healthy social relationships poses substantial societal and economic burdens in the future.

Social media can be an invaluable tool for keeping you in touch with friends, loved ones, and the broader world at this time of social distancing and isolation. But be mindful of how it makes you feel. Excessive use can fuel feelings of anxiety, depression, isolation, and FOMO (fear of missing out). If spending time on social media exacerbates your stress, anxiety, and uncertainty, take steps to limit your engagement.

The results of a 2014 study suggested a connection between social networking sites (SNS) and mental health issues, such as depressive symptoms, changes in self-esteem, and internet addiction. Exceptions would be, of course, flooding or a volcanic eruption in your immediate vicinity. Once the apparent threat is perceived, whether it is real and present, it will start the physiological survival process in the body.

There is a fine line between being well informed and being oversaturated. We would all be better off if we could decrease our exposure to the fear-based and negative messages of the news of the day. We would be a lot less paranoid. Recently, there has been a lot of fake news to top it all. It is not always easy to tell the difference between fake news and factual news. As for me, since 9/11, I have limited my news exposure, whether from my TV, my computer, or my phone. I am very protective of my mental and emotional energy.

 A lifetime exposure of minute doses of toxins is very harmful to your health.

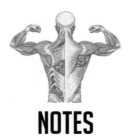

NOTES

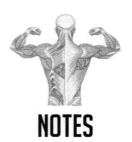

NOTES

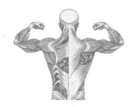

BOOK 1 SUMMARY HIGHLIGHTS

Chapter 1: In epigenetics, your gene expression is 100 percent within your control.

Chapter 2: Pain is a friendly messenger. Self-healing is holistic and relies on you to provide the healthy raw materials and the right environment for healing.

Chapter 3: Most degenerative diseases have two basic mechanisms: congestion and depletion.

Chapter 4: A lifetime exposure of minute doses of toxins is very harmful to your health.

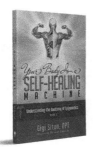
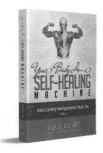

Now that you have laid a good groundwork on what is epigenetics, I am sure you are ready to learn more. Book Two, *The Anatomy of Epigenetics*, and Book Three, *How Epigenetics Heals You*, will systematically build momentum on your foundational knowledge of epigenetics.

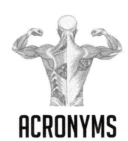

ACRONYMS

ACERO	Aberdeen Centre for Energy Regulation and Obesity
ADD	Attention Deficit Disorder
ADHD	Attention Deficit Hyperactivity Disorder
AGD	Anogenital Distance
AFO	Animal Feeding Operations
ALA	Alpha Linolenic Acid
AM	Amplitude Modulation
ANS	Autonomic Nervous System
ARA	Adenine Arabinoside
ATP	Adenosine Triphosphate
BAP	British Association of Psychopharmacology
BALT	Bronchial-associated Lymphoid Tissue
BBM	Buteyko Breathing Medicine
BBT	Buteyko Breathing Technique
BHA	Butylated Hydroxyanisole
BHT	Butylated Hydroxytoluene
BPA	Bisphenol A
CAFOS	Confined Animal Feeding Operations
CCK	Cholecystokinin
CD	Celiac Disease
CDC	Centers for Disease Control and Prevention

CKD	Cyclic Ketogenic Diet
CLA	Conjugated Linoleic Acid
COPD	Chronic Obstructive Pulmonary Disease
CSF	Cerebrospinal Fluid
CST	Craniosacral Therapy
CT	Computer Tomography
DGLA	Dihomogamma-Linolenic Acid
DNA	Deoxyribonucleic Acid
DH	Dermatitis Herpetiformis
DHA	Docosahexaenoic Acid
DSM	Diagnostic and Statistical Manual of Mental Disorders
ECG	Electrocardiogram
ECT	Electroconvulsive Therapy
ED	Erectile Dysfunction
EGF	Epidermal Growth Factor
EMG	Electromyograph
EMF	Electromagnetic Field
EPA	Environmental Protection Agency
EPA	Eicosapentaenoic Acid
EWG	Environmental Working Group
FAO	Food and Agriculture Organization of the United Nations
FDA	Food and Drug Administration
FM	Frequency Modulation
FPG	Fasting Plasma Glucose
GABA	Gamma-Aminobutyric Acid
GALT	Gut-Associated Lymphoid Tissue
GERD	Gastroesophageal Reflux Disease
GLA	Gamma Linolenic Acid

GMO	Genetically Modified Organism
HDL	High Density Lipoproteins
HMP	Human Microbiome Project
HPKD	High Protein Ketogenic Diet
IBS	Irritable Bowel Syndrome
IF	Intermittent Fasting
IGF	Insulin-like Growth Factor
IM	Innovative Medicine
LDL	Low Density Lipoproteins
MCT	Medium Chain Triglyceride
MnSOD	Manganese-dependent Superoxide Dismutase
MRSA	Methicillin-Resistant Staphylococcus Aureus
MS	Multiple Sclerosis
mV	milliVolts
NASA	National Aeronautics and Space Administration
NAFLD	Nonalcoholic Fatty Liver Disease
NCGS	Nonceliac Gluten Sensitivity
NIH	National Institutes of Health
NLFES	Nonionizing Low Frequency Electromagnetic Waves
NM	Neural Manipulation
NSAIDs	Nonsteroidal Anti-inflammatory Drugs
OTC	Over The Counter
PCOS	Polycystic Ovary Syndrome
PDE	Phosphodiesterase
PEFR	Peak Respiratory Flow Rate
PENI	Psychoendocrinoimmunology
PFOA	Perflourooctanoic Acid
PNEI	Psychoneuroendocrinoimmunology
PNI	Psychoneuroimmunology
PPI	Proton Pump Inhibitors

PT	Physical Therapy
PTH	Parathyroid Hormone
PTSD	Post-Traumatic Stress Disorder
RBC	Red Blood Cell
rBGH	Recombinant Bovine Growth Hormone
REM	Rapid Eye Movement
RNA	Ribonucleic Acid
ROM	Range of Motion
ROS	Reactive Oxygen Species
SAD	Seasonal Affective Disorder
SAM	Sulfur-adenosylmethionine dismutase
SCN	Suprachiasmatic Nucleus
SIAM	Italian Society of Andrology and Sexual Medicine
SKD	Standard Ketogenic Diet
SLES	Sodium Laureth Sulfate
SLS	Sodium Lauryl Sulfate
TBHQ	Tertiary Butylhydroquinone
TCM	Traditional Chinese Medicine
TEA	Triethanomaline
TKD	Targeted Ketogenic Diet
UHT	Ultra-heat Treated
USDA	United States Department of Agriculture
UTHSC	University of Tennessee Health Science Center
VM	Visceral Manipulation
VRA	Vancomycin-resistant Enterococcus
WBC	White Blood Cell
WHO	World Health Organization
XEs	Xenoestrogens

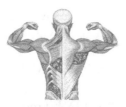

REFERENCES

1   Rachel Rettner, Epigenetics:Definition and Examples; June 24, 2013, https://www.livescience.com/37703-epigenetics.html

2   Michael Skinner, PhD, "Unified Theory of Evolution," Published by Aeon on: 9th November 2016, https://aeon.co/essays/on-epigenetics-we-need-both-darwin-s-and-lamarck-s-theories

3   Zirkle, Conway (1935). "The Inheritance of Acquired Characters and the Provisional Hypothesis of Pangenesis," The American Naturalist. 69 (724): 417–445. doi:10.1086/280617.

4   Barthélemy-Madaule, Madeleine (1982). Lamarck, the Mythical Precursor: A Study of the Relations Between Science and Ideology. English translation by M. H. Shank. MIT Press. ISBN 978-0-262-02179-1.

5   Nilsson EE, Sadler-Riggleman I, Skinner MK. Environmentally induced epigenetic transgenerational inheritance of disease. Environ Epigenet. 2018;4(2):dvy016. Published 2018 Jul 17. doi:10.1093/eep/dvy016

6   Burdge GC, Lillycrop KA. Fatty acids and epigenetics. Curr Opin Clin Nutr Metab Care. 2014 Mar;17(2):156-61. doi: 10.1097/MCO.0000000000000023. PMID: 24322369.

7   Heo JB, Sung S. Encoding memory of winter by noncoding RNAs. Epigenetics. 2011 May;6(5):544-7. doi: 10.4161/epi.6.5.15235. Epub 2011 May 1. PMID: 21406964.

8   Zucchi FC, Yao Y, Metz GA. The secret language of destiny: stress imprinting and transgenerational origins of disease. Front Genet. 2012;3:96. Published 2012 Jun 4. doi:10.3389/fgene.2012.00096

9   Michael K. Skinner, Environmental Epigenetics and a Unified Theory of the Molecular Aspects of Evolution: A Neo-Lamarckian Concept

that Facilitates Neo-Darwinian Evolution, Genome Biology and Evolution, Volume 7, Issue 5, May 2015, Pages 1296–1302, https://doi.org/10.1093/gbe/evv073

10   Christopher W Kuzawa & Zaneta M Thayer, Timescales of human adaptation: the role of epigenetic processes, EPIGENOMICS VOL. 3, NO. 2 PERSPECTIVE Free Access, Published Online:20 Apr 2011https://doi.org/10.2217/epi.11.11

11   Alegría-Torres JA, Baccarelli A, Bollati V. Epigenetics, and lifestyle. Epigenomics. 2011;3(3):267-277. doi:10.2217/epi.11.22

12   Suchy FJ et.al.; NIH Consensus and State-of-the-science Statements, 31 Jan 2010, 27(2):1-27 PMID: 20186234

13   Christina Mattina, Filipino Americans Over 50 at High Risk of Diabetes, Even If Not Obese. April 21, 2017, https://www.ajmc.com/newsroom/filipino-americans-over-50-at-high-risk-of-diabetes-even-if-not-obese

14   Gustafson C. Bruce Lipton, PhD: The Jump From Cell Culture to Consciousness. Integr Med (Encinitas). 2017;16(6):44-50.

15   https://www.cdc.gov/drugoverdose/epidemic/index.html

16   James M. DuBois, et. al, 18 Dec 2017"; Exploring Unnecessary Invasive Procedures In The United States: A Retrospective Mixed-Methods Analysis Of Cases From 2008-2016;" https://www.ncbi.nlm.nih.gov/pmc/articles/PMC5735893/

17   Stahel PF, VanderHeiden TF, Kim FJ. Why do surgeons continue to perform unnecessary surgery? Patient Saf Surg. 2017; 11:1. Published 2017 Jan 13. doi:10.1186/s13037-016-0117-6

18   Global patient outcomes after elective surgery: prospective cohort study in 27 low-, middle- and high-income countries. BJA: British Journal of Anaesthesia, Volume 117, Issue 5, 1 November 2016, Pages 601–609, https://doi.org/10.1093/bja/aew316

19   "Death by Medicine" from www.mercola.com

20   Fowle, Farnsworth (July 26, 1976). "Henry K. Beecher, Doctor in Boston – Won World Fame for Work in Anesthesia and Ethics." The New York Times. p. 26. Retrieved August 25, 2009.

21   Beecher HK. The powerful placebo. J Am Med Assoc. 1955 Dec 24;159(17):1602-6.

22   Munnangi S, Angus LD. Placebo Effect. [Updated 2020 Feb 18]. In: StatPearls [Internet]. Treasure Island (FL): StatPearls Publishing; 2020 Jan. Available from: https://www.ncbi.nlm.nih.gov/books/NBK513296/

23 Ted J Kaptchuk, et. al.; "Sham device v inert pill: randomised controlled trial of two placebo treatments" BMJ 2006; doi: https://doi.org/10.1136/bmj.38726.603310.55 (Published 01 February 2006) Cite this as: BMJ 2006; bmj; bmj.38726.603310.55vl

24 Colagiuri B, Schenk LA, Kessler MD, Dorsey SG, Colloca L. The placebo effect: From concepts to genes. Neuroscience. 2015 Oct 29; 307:171-90.

25 Beecher HK. The powerful placebo. J Am Med Assoc 1955;159:17:1602-6

26 Leucht, S., Helfer, B., Gartlehner, G. et al. How effective are common medications: a perspective based on meta-analyses of major drugs. BMC Med 13, 253 (2015). https://doi.org/10.1186/s12916-015-0494-1

27 Tinetti ME, Han L, Lee DS, et al. Antihypertensive medications and serious fall injuries in a nationally representative sample of older adults. JAMA Intern Med. 2014;174(4):588-595. doi:10.1001/jamainternmed.2013.14764

28 Musini VM, Tejani AM, Bassett K, Wright JM. Pharmacotherapy for hypertension in the elderly. Cochrane Database Syst Rev. 2009;(4):CD000028. Published 2009 Oct 7. doi:10.1002/14651858.CD000028.pub2

29 Tjia J, Velten SJ, Parsons C, Valluri S, Briesacher BA. Studies to reduce unnecessary medication use in frail older adults: a systematic review. Drugs Aging. 2013;30(5):285-307. doi:10.1007/s40266-013-0064-1

30 Maher RL, Hanlon J, Hajjar ER. Clinical consequences of polypharmacy in elderly. Expert Opin Drug Saf. 2014;13(1):57-65. doi:10.1517/14740338.2013.827660

31 Tjia J, Velten SJ, Parsons C, Valluri S, Briesacher BA. Studies to reduce unnecessary medication use in frail older adults: a systematic review. Drugs Aging. 2013;30(5):285-307. doi:10.1007/s40266-013-0064-1

32 Bourgeois FT, Shannon MW, Valim C, et al. Adverse drug events in the outpatient setting: an 11-year national analysis. Pharmacoepidemiol Drug Saf. 2010;19:901–10

33 Bourgeois FT, Shannon MW, Valim C, et al. Adverse drug events in the outpatient setting: an 11-year national analysis. Pharmacoepidemiol Drug Saf. 2010;19:901–10.

34 Hohl CM, Dankoff J, Colacone A, et al. Polypharmacy, adverse drug-related events, and potential adverse drug interactions in elderly patients presenting to an emergency department. Ann Emerg Med. 2001;38:666–71

35 Doan J, Zakrewski-Jakubiak H, Roy J, et al. Prevalence and risk of potential cytochrome p450-mediated drug-drug interactions in older hospitalized patients with polypharmacy. Ann Pharmacother. 2013;47:324–32

36 Magaziner J, Cadigan DA, Fedder DO, Hebel JR. Medication use and functional decline among community-dwelling older women. J Aging Health. 1989;1:470–484.

37 Martin NJ, Stones MJ, Young JE, et al. Development of delirium: a prospective cohort study in a community hospital. International Psychogeriatrics. 2000;12:117–27.

38 Jyrkka J, Enlund H, Lavikainen P, et al. Association of polypharmacy with nutritional status, functional ability and cognitive capacity over a three-year period in an elderly population. Pharmacoepidemiol Drug Saf. 2010;20:514–522.

39 Heuberger RA, Caudell K. Polypharmacy and nutritional status in older adults. Drugs Aging. 2011;28:315–323.

40 Fletcher PC, Berg K, Dalby DM, Hirdes JP. Risk factors for falling among community-based seniors. J Patient Saf. 2009;5:61–66.

41 "Americans Taking More Prescription Drugs Than Ever." Centers for Disease Control and Prevention. 19 Jan. 2017.

42 Holland EG, Degury FV. Drug induced disorders. American Family Physician. 1997:56:1781-8. 1791-2

43 Hall MJ, Schwartzman A, Zhang J, Liu X. Ambulatory Surgery Data From Hospitals and Ambulatory Surgery Centers: United States, 2010. Natl Health Stat Report. 2017;(102):1-15.

44 Hedegaard H, Miniño AM, Warner M. Drug Overdose Deaths in the United States, 1999–2018.pdf icon NCHS Data Brief, no 356. Hyattsville, MD: National Center for Health Statistics. 2020.

45 Baer HA. The sociopolitical status of U.S. naturopathy at the dawn of the 21st century. Med Anthropol Q. 2001;15(3):329-346. doi:10.1525/maq.2001.15.3.329

46 Allen, Frederick M. (January 1923). "Clinical observations with insulin." University of Toronto Libraries: The Discovery and Early

Development of Insulin. Morristown, NJ: Journal of Metabolic Research.

47 "The Cost of Diabetes," https://www.diabetes.org/resources/statistics/cost-diabetes

48 Equine Podiatry, 2007, 'Pain Receptor', https://www.sciencedirect.com/topics/immunology-and-microbiology/pain-receptor

49 Jean-Pierre Barral D.O., Understanding the Message of Your Body, North Atlantic Books, November 2007

50 https://www.barralinstitute.com/docs/articles/stlwj-the-messages-of-your-body.pdf

51 Wetzler G, Roland M, Fryer-Dietz S, Dettmann-Ahern D. CranioSacral Therapy and Visceral Manipulation: A New Treatment Intervention for Concussion Recovery. Med Acupunct. 2017;29(4):239-248. doi:10.1089/acu.2017.1222

52 Dr. Lisa Metzgar, PhD; "Let's All Eat Dirt?!?": https://www.epicorimmune.com/blog/2017/10/16/lets-all-eat-dirt

53 Alexandre-Silva, Gabriel M.; Brito-Souza, Pablo A.; Oliveira, Ana C.S.; Cerni, Felipe A.; Zottich, Umberto; Pucca, Manuela B. (December 2018). "The hygiene hypothesis at a glance: Early exposures, immune mechanism and novel therapies." Acta Tropica. 188: 16–26. doi:10.1016/j.actatropica.2018.08.032

54 Bloomfield SF, Stanwell-Smith R, Crevel RW, Pickup J. Too clean, or not too clean: the hygiene hypothesis and home hygiene. Clin Exp Allergy. 2006;36(4):402-425. doi:10.1111/j.1365-2222.2006.02463.x

55 http://www.pbs.org/wgbh/evolution/library/10/4/l_104_07.html

56 https://www.radiologyinfo.org/en/info.cfm?pg=nerveblock

57 Emanuele Rinninella, Pauline Raoul, Marco Cintoni, Francesco Franceschi, Giacinto Abele Donato Miggiano, Antonio Gasbarrini, and Maria Cristina Mele1," What is the Healthy Gut Microbiota Composition? A Changing Ecosystem across Age, Environment, Diet, and Diseases"; https://www.ncbi.nlm.nih.gov/pmc/articles/PMC6351938/

58 "Circadian Rhythms"; https://www.nigms.nih.gov/education/fact-sheets/Pages/circadian-rhythms.aspx

59 Anthony H Tsang, Johanna L Barclay, and Henrik Oster, "Interactions between endocrine and circadian systems"; in Journal of Molecular Endocrinology; https://jme.bioscientifica.com/view/journals/jme/52/1/R1.xml

60 Rahul Mittal et.al., "Neurotransmitters: The critical modulators regulating gut-brain axis"; https://www.ncbi.nlm.nih.gov/pmc/articles/PMC5772764/

61 "Lack of Sleep Increases Your Risk of Some Cancers"; https://www.sleepfoundation.org/articles/lack-sleep-increases-your-risk-some-cancers

62 "Sleep deprivation leads to symptoms of schizophrenia"; https://www.uni-bonn.de/Press-releases/sleep-deprivation-leads-to-symptoms-of-schizophrenia

63 "Eating for Health: A Medical Doctor's Program for Conquering Disease" book by Dr. J Fuhrman - 1998 – Macmillan; and Hereward Carrington, PhD, "Fasting for Health and Long Life" book;

64 Shanthi Johnson & Krista Leck; "The Effects of Dietary Fasting on Physical Balance Among Healthy Young Women"; https://nutritionj.biomedcentral.com/articles/10.1186/1475-2891-9-18?optIn=false

65 Angus Stewart; Senior Lecturer in Nutrition and Dietetics, Edith Cowan University; "Health Check: 'Food Comas,' Or Why Eating Sometimes Makes You Sleepy"; September 21, 2015; https://theconversation.com/health-check-food-comas-or-why-eating-sometimes-makes-you-sleepy-44355

66 Poplawski MM, Mastaitis JW, Yang XJ, Mobbs CV. Hypothalamic responses to fasting indicate metabolic reprogramming away from glycolysis toward lipid oxidation. Endocrinology. 2010;151(11):5206-5217. doi:10.1210/en.2010-0702

67 Almeneessier AS, BaHammam AS. How does diurnal intermittent fasting impact sleep, daytime sleepiness, and markers of the biological clock? Current insights. Nat Sci Sleep. 2018;10:439-452. Published 2018 Dec 7. doi:10.2147/NSS.S165637

68 Nicole K Valtorta, Mona Kanaan, Simon Gilbody, Sara Ronzi, Barbara Hanratty; "Loneliness and social isolation as risk factors for coronary heart disease and stroke: systematic review and meta-analysis of longitudinal observational studies;" https://heart.bmj.com/content/102/13/1009

69 Willett W. C. Balancing Lifestyle and Genomics Research for Disease Prevention. Science. 2002; 296:695–98

70 Janelle KC1, Barr SI.; J Am Diet Assoc. 1995 Feb;95(2):180-6, 189, quiz 187-8. Nutrient intakes and eating behavior scores of

vegetarian and nonvegetarian women.; https://www.ncbi.nlm.nih.gov/pubmed/7852684

71 Roman Pawlak, Scott James Parrott, Sudha Raj, Diana Cullum-Dugan, Debbie Lucus; "How prevalent is vitamin B12 deficiency among vegetarians?"; https://academic.oup.com/nutritionreviews/article/71/2/110/1940320

72 https://www.britannica.com/science/traditional-Chinese-medicine

73 Giovanni Musso, Carla Olivetti, Maurizio Cassader, Roberto Gambino;" Obstructive Sleep Apnea–Hypopnea Syndrome and Nonalcoholic Fatty Liver Disease: Emerging Evidence and Mechanisms"; Semin Liver Dis 2012; 32(01): 049-064; DOI: 10.1055/s-0032-1306426; https://www.thieme-connect.com/products/ejournals/html/10.1055/s-0032-1306426

74 M. Gerson, "The cure of advanced cancer by diet therapy: A summary of 30 years of clinical experimentation." PhysiolChem. Phys., 10,449(1978).

75 Mark P.Mattson, RuiqianWan;" Beneficial effects of intermittent fasting and caloric restriction on the cardiovascular and cerebrovascular systems", https://www.sciencedirect.com/science/article/abs/pii/S095528630400261X#!

76 Mario C. De Tullio, Ph.D. (Department of Plant Biology and Pathology, University of Bari) © 2010 Nature Education; "The Mystery of Vitamin C", Citation: De Tullio, M. C. (2010) The Mystery of Vitamin C. Nature Education 3(9):48; https://www.nature.com/scitable/topicpage/the-mystery-of-vitamin-c-14167861/

77 Mozaffari H, et.al.;"Dietary fat, saturated fatty acid, and monounsaturated fatty acid intakes and risk of bone fracture: a systematic review and meta-analysis of observational studies." Osteoporos Int. 2018 Sep;29(9):1949-1961. doi: 10.1007/s00198-018-4540-7. Epub 2018 Jun 12.; https://www.ncbi.nlm.nih.gov/pubmed/29947872

78 Sylvia Christakos, et.al. "Vitamin D and Intestinal Calcium Absorption"; Published online 2011 Jun 1. doi: 10.1016/j.mce.2011.05.038; https://www.ncbi.nlm.nih.gov/pmc/articles/PMC3405161/

79 The importance of good hydration for the prevention of chronic diseases. Manz F, Wentz A Nutr Rev. 2005 Jun; Review 63(6 Pt 2): S2-5.

80 Hou L, Zhang X, Wang D, Baccarelli A. Environmental chemical exposures, and human epigenetics. Int J Epidemiol. 2012;41(1):79-105. doi:10.1093/ije/dyr154

81 Yun MJ, Kang DM, Lee KH, Kim YK, Kim JE. Multiple chemical sensitivity caused by exposure to ignition coal fumes: a case report. Ann Occup Environ Med. 2013;25(1):32. Published 2013 Nov 1. doi:10.1186/2052-4374-25-32

82 Developmental origin of chronic diseases: toxicological implication. Bezek S, Ujházy E, Mach M, Navarová J, Dubovický M Interdiscip Toxicol. 2008 Jun; 1(1):29-31.

83 Hou L, Zhang X, Wang D, Baccarelli A. Environmental chemical exposures and human epigenetics. Int J Epidemiol. 2012;41(1):79-105. doi:10.1093/ije/dyr154

84 https://gmoanswers.com/get-know-gmos-month-science-gmos

85 Mesnage R, Clair E, Gress S, Then C, Székács A, Séralini GE. Cytotoxicity on human cells of Cry1Ab and Cry1Ac Bt insecticidal toxins alone or with a glyphosate-based herbicide. J Appl Toxicol. 2013;33(7):695-699. doi:10.1002/jat.2712

86 United States Environmental Protection Agency. "DDT – A Brief History and Status." EPA, (n.d.). Retrieved May 28, 2019, from https://www.epa.gov/ingredients-used-pesticide-products/ddt-brief-history-and-status

87 A. J. Cessna, , A. L. Darwent, , K. J. Kirkland, , L. Townley-Smith, K. N. Harker, and , L. P. Lefkovitch; Residues of glyphosate and its metabolite AMPA in wheat seed and foliage following preharvest applications ;Canadian Journal of Plant Science, 1994, 74(3): 653-661, https://doi.org/10.4141/cjps94-117

88 Velimirov A, Binter C, Zentek J, "Biological effects of transgenic maize NK603xMON810 fed in long term reproduction studies in mice." November 2008

89 Hilbeck, A., Binimelis, R., Defarge, N. et al. "No scientific consensus on GMO safety." Environ Sci Eur 27, 4 (2015). https://doi.org/10.1186/s12302-014-0034-1

90 Lustig, R.H., Schmidt, L.A., & Brindis, C.D. (2012, February 2). Public health: The toxic truth about sugar. Nature, 487(5), 27-29. doi:10.1038/482027a. Retrieved from http://www.nature.com/nature/journal/v482/n7383/full/482027a.html

91 Akula Nookaraju, et.al., "Molecular Approaches for Enhancing Sweetness In Fruits And Vegetables." November 2010; Scientia Horticulturae 127(1):1–15, https://www.researchgate.net/publication/257147774_Molecular_approaches_for_enhancing_sweetness_in_fruits_and_vegetables

92 Fournet M, Bonté F, Desmoulière A. Glycation Damage: A Possible Hub for Major Pathophysiological Disorders and Aging. Aging Dis. 2018;9(5):880-900. Published 2018 Oct 1. doi:10.14336/AD.2017.1121

93 Adewale Fadaka, Basiru Ajiboye, Oluwafemi Ojo, Olusola Adewale, Israel Olayide, Rosemary Emuowhochere, Biology of glucose metabolization in cancer cells, Journal of Oncological Sciences, Volume 3, Issue 2, 2017, Pages 45-51, ISSN 2452-3364, https://doi.org/10.1016/j.jons.2017.06.002.

94 Linda Rath, "Cancer and Sugar: Is There a Link?", https://www.webmd.com/cancer/features/cancer-sugar-link#1

95 Whitehouse CR, Boullata J, McCauley LA. The potential toxicity of artificial sweeteners. AAOHN J. 2008;56(6):251-261. doi:10.3928/08910162-20080601-02

96 https://www.canada.ca/en/health-canada/services/food-nutrition/food-safety/food-additives/sugar-substitutes/information-document-proposal-reinstate-saccharin-use-sweetener-foods-canada.html, extracted October30, 2020

97 Leonard MM, Vasagar B. US perspective on gluten-related diseases. Clin Exp Gastroenterol. 2014; 7:25-37. Published 2014 Jan 24. doi:10.2147/CEG.S54567

98 Volta U, Caio G, Tovoli F, De Giorgio R (2013). "Non-celiac gluten sensitivity: questions still to be answered despite increasing awareness." Cellular and Molecular Immunology (Review). 10 (5): 383–392. doi:10.1038/cmi.2013.2

99 Tovoli F, Masi C, Guidetti E, Negrini G, Paterini P, Bolondi L (Mar 16, 2015)." Clinical and diagnostic aspects of gluten related disorders." World J Clin Cases (Review). 3 (3): 275–84. doi:10.12998/wjcc.v3.i3.275

100 Volta U, Caio G, Tovoli F, De Giorgio R (September 2013). "Non-celiac gluten sensitivity: questions still to be answered despite increasing awareness." Cellular & Molecular Immunology (Review). 10 (5): 383–92. doi:10.1038/cmi.2013.28

101 Katherine Czapp. "Putting the Polish on Those Humble Beans.", https://www.westonaprice.org/health-topics/food-features/putting-the-polish-on-those-humble-beans/

102 Arnold LE, Lofthouse N, Hurt E. Artificial food colors and attention-deficit/hyperactivity symptoms: conclusions to dye for. Neurotherapeutics. 2012;9(3):599-609. doi:10.1007/s13311-012-0133-x

103 Mohamed M. Hashem1, et.al.,"Toxicological Impact of Amaranth, Sunset Yellow and Curcumin as Food Coloring Agents in Albino Rats." https://www.jpmsonline.com/wp-content/uploads/2011/04/JPMS-VOL1-ISSUE2-PAGES43-51-OA.pdf

104 Pamela L. Horn-Ross, Esther M. John, Alison J. Canchola, Susan L. Stewart, Marion M. Lee, Phytoestrogen Intake and Endometrial Cancer Risk, JNCI: Journal of the National Cancer Institute, Volume 95, Issue 15, 6 August 2003, Pages 1158–1164, https://doi.org/10.1093/jnci/djg015

105 Duffy, C., Perez, K. and Partridge, A. (2007), Implications of Phytoestrogen Intake for Breast Cancer. CA: A Cancer Journal for Clinicians, 57: 260-277. doi:10.3322/CA.57.5.260

106 The WHO Recommended Classification of Pesticides by Hazard and Guidelines to Classification 2000-2002. Geneva, World Health Organization, 2002.

107 Liu J, Schelar E. Pesticide exposure and child neurodevelopment: summary and implications. Workplace Health Saf. 2012;60(5):235-243. doi:10.1177/216507991206000507

108 USDA, Pesticide Data Program 2015

109 Elke Kennepohl, James S. Bus et.al., in Hayes' Handbook of Pesticide Toxicology (Third Edition), 2010 "Phenoxy Herbicides (2,4-D)"; https://www.sciencedirect.com/topics/agricultural-and-biological-sciences/phenoxy-herbicide

110 Marina M. Vdovenko, Alexandra S. Stepanova, Sergei A. Eremin, Nguyen Van Cuong, Natalia A. Uskova, Ivan Yu Sakharov, Quantification of 2,4-dichlorophenoxyacetic acid in oranges and mandarins by chemiluminescent ELISA, Food Chemistry, Volume 141, Issue 2,2013, Pages 865-868, ISSN 0308-8146, https://doi.org/10.1016/j.foodchem.2013.04.060.

111 Understanding Concentrated Animal Feeding Operations and Their Impact on Communities.

112 https://en.wikipedia.org/wiki/Concentrated_animal_feeding_ operation

113 "Animal Feeding Operations." United States Department of Agriculture

114 de Albuquerque Fernandes, S.A., Magnavita, A.P.A., Ferrao, S.P.B. et al. Daily ingestion of tetracycline residue present in pasteurized milk: a public health problem. Environ Sci Pollut Res 21, 3427– 3434 (2014). https://doi.org/10.1007/s11356-013-2286-5

115 Sozańska B. Raw Cow's Milk and Its Protective Effect on Allergies and Asthma. Nutrients. 2019;11(2):469. Published 2019 Feb 22. doi:10.3390/nu11020469

116 Natasha Longo; "9 Reasons To Stop Drinking Any Kind of Pasteurized Milk" ttps://www.preventdisease.com/news/ 14/070314_9-Reasons-Stop-Drinking-Pasteurized-Milk.shtml

117 Alessandra Bordoni, et.al."Dairy products and inflammation: A review of the clinical evidence."; https://www.tandfonline.com/doi/citedby/1 0.1080/10408398.2014.967385?scroll=top&needAccess=true

118 Gottlieb S. Early exposure to cows' milk raises risk of diabetes in high risk children. BMJ. 2000;321(7268):1040. https://www.ncbi. nlm.nih.gov/pmc/articles/PMC1173447/

119 Nekouei O, VanLeeuwen J, Sanchez J, Kelton D, Tiwari A, Keefe G. Herd-level risk factors for infection with bovine leukemia virus in Canadian dairy herds. Prev Vet Med. 2015;119(3-4):105-113. doi: 10.1016/j.prevetmed.2015.02.025

120 https://www.agweb.com/article/a-look-at-johnes-disease-NAA- university-news-release

121 "Case-Control Study of Risk Factors for Hip Fractures in the Elderly." American Journal of Epidemiology. Vol. 139, No. 5, 1994

122 Colditz GA, Philpott SE, Hankinson SE. The Impact of the Nurses' Health Study on Population Health: Prevention, Translation, and Control. Am J Public Health. 2016;106(9):1540-1545. doi:10.2105/ AJPH.2016.303343

123 April Mccarthy; "FDA Concedes Antibiotic Use In Farm Animals Must Be Phased Out."; https://www.preventdisease. com/news/13/121213_FDA-Concedes-Antibiotic-Use-In-Farm- Animals-Must-Be-Phased-Out.shtml

124 www.fda.gov

125 Choi AL, Zhang Y, Sun G, et al. Association of lifetime exposure to fluoride and cognitive functions in Chinese children: a pilot study [published correction appears in Neurotoxicol Teratol. 2015 Sep-Oct;51():89]. Neurotoxicol Teratol. 2015; 47:96-101. doi: 10.1016/j.ntt.2014.11.001

126 Röösli M. Radiofrequency electromagnetic field exposure and non-specific symptoms of ill health: a systematic review. Environ Res. 2008;107(2):277-287. doi:10.1016/j.envres.2008.02.003

127 Effect of radiofrequency radiation from Wi-Fi devices on mercury release from amalgam restorations Maryam Paknahad, S. M. J. Mortazavi, Shoaleh Shahidi, Ghazal Mortazavi, Masoud Haghani Environ Health Sci Eng. 2016; 14: 12. Published online 2016 Jul 13. doi: 10.1186/s40201-016-0253-z PMCID: PMC4944481

128 https://charlottenaturalwellness.com/2015/04/01/3-common-things-that-wreck-your-thyroid/

129 The Hidden Danger of Chlorine in our Bath Water. http://ezinearticles.com/?The-Hidden-Danger-Of-Chlorine-In-Our-Bath-Water&id=71857. Andie Klein.

130 Morris RD. Drinking water and cancer. Environ Health Perspect. 1995;103 Suppl 8(Suppl 8):225-231. doi:10.1289/ehp.95103s8225

131 Agency for Toxic Substances and Disease Registry. Medical Management Guidelines (MMGs) for Chlorine (Cl2). Atlanta, GA: Agency for Toxic Substances and Disease Registry, Division of Toxicology; 2004.

132 IARC Monographs on the Evaluation of Carcinogenic Risks to Humans vol. 17 (Paris: International Agency for Research on Cancer), vol. 40 (1986).

133 Study on Enhancing the Endocrine Disrupter Priority List with a Focus on Low Production Volume Chemicals, Revised Report to DG Environment (Hersholm, Denmark: DHI Water and Environment, 2007), http://ec.europa.eu/environment/endocrine/documents/final_report_2007.pdf

134 https://en.wikipedia.org/wiki/Tert-Butylhydroquinone

135 Yuan GF, Sun B, Yuan J, Wang QM. Effects of different cooking methods on health-promoting compounds of broccoli. J Zhejiang Univ Sci B. 2009;10(8):580-588. doi:10.1631/jzus.B0920051

136 Xiang, Shuyu and Zou, et al., February 2020, Effects of microwave heating on the protein structure, digestion properties, and Maillard

products of gluten}, V 57, Journal of Food Science and Technology, doi 10.1007/s13197-020-04249-0

137 Nemethy M, Clore ER. Microwave heating of infant formula and breast milk. J Pediatr Health Care. 1990;4(3):131-135. doi:10.1016/0891-5245(90)90050-g

138 Jose-Luis Sagripanti & Mays L. Swicord (1986) DNA Structural Changes Caused by Microwave Radiation, International Journal of Radiation Biology and Related Studies in Physics, Chemistry and Medicine, 50:1, 47-50, DOI: 10.1080/09553008614550431

139 Riquet AM, Breysse C, Dahbi L, Loriot C, Severin I, Chagnon MC. The consequences of physical post-treatments (microwave and electron-beam) on food/packaging interactions: A physicochemical and toxicological approach. Food Chem. 2016;199:59-69. doi:10.1016/j.foodchem.2015.09.034

140 National Center for Biotechnology Information. PubChem Database. Caffeine, CID=2519, https://pubchem.ncbi.nlm.nih. gov/compound/Caffeine (accessed on July 14, 2020)

141 Bhattacharya, S. K., Satyan, K. S., & Chakrabarti, A. (1997). Anxiogenic action of caffeine: an experimental study in rats. Journal of Psychopharmacology, 11(3), 219–224. https://doi. org/10.1177/026988119701100304

142 Human health effects of air pollution; MarilenaKampa, EliasCastanas; https://doi.org/10.1016/j.envpol.2007.06.012; Air Pollution and Human Health; By Lester B. Lave, Eugene P. Seskin

143 Air pollution: mechanisms of neuroinflammation and CNS disease; Michelle L. Block1LilianCalderón-Garcidueñas; Trends in Neurosciences, Volume 32, Issue 9, September 2009, Pages 506-516; https://doi.org/10.1016/j.tins.2009.05.009

144 Edwin J. Routledge; et al. (1998). "Some alkyl hydroxy benzoate preservatives (parabens) are estrogenic" Toxicol Appl Pharmacol. 1998 Nov;153(1):12-9

145 Hauser R, Calafat AM. Phthalates, and human health. Occup. Environ. Med. 2005;62(11):806–818.

146 NRC. Phthalates and Cumulative Risk Assessment: The Tasks Ahead. Washington, DC: The National Academies Press; 2008

147 Gray LE Jr., Ostby J, Furr J, Price M, Veeramachaneni DN, Parks L. Perinatal exposure to the phthalates DEHP, BBP, and DINP, but not DEP, DMP, or DOTP, alters sexual differentiation of the male rat.

Toxicol. Sci. 2000;58(2):350–365.; Foster PM, Mylchreest E, Gaido KW, Sar M. Effects of phthalate esters on the developing reproductive tract of male rats. Hum. Reprod. Update. 2001;7(3):231–235.; Fisher JS, Macpherson S, Marchetti N, Sharpe RM. Human "testicular dysgenesis syndrome": A possible model using in-utero exposure of the rat to dibutyl phthalate. Hum. Reprod. 2003;18(7):1383–1394.

148 Fennell TR, Krol WL, Sumner SC, Snyder RW. Pharmacokinetics of dibutyl phthalate in pregnant rats. Toxicol. Sci. 2004;82(2):407–418

149 Silva MJ, Reidy JA, Herbert AR, Preau JL, Needham LL, Calafat AM. Detection of phthalate metabolites in human aminiotic fluid. Bull. Environ. Contam. Toxicol. 2004;72(6):1226–1231.

150 Citation: Klöting N, Hesselbarth N, Gericke M, Kunath A, Biemann R, Chakaroun R, et al. (2015) Di-(2-Ethylhexyl)-Phthalate (DEHP) Causes Impaired Adipocyte Function and Alters Serum Metabolites. PLoS ONE 10(12): e0143190. https://doi.org/10.1371/journal.pone.0143190

151 Green K., Cheeks L., Chapman J.M. (1987) Surfactant Pharmacokinetics in the Eye. In: Saettone M.F., Bucci M., Speiser P. (eds) Ophthalmic Drug Delivery. FIDIA Research Series, vol 11. Springer, New York, NY

152 WHO. ILO. International Chemical Safety Card for Sodium Lauryl Sulfate (ICSC 0502). Aug 1997. http://www.ilo.org/legacy/english/protection/safework/cis/products/icsc/dtasht/_icsc05/icsc0502.htm

153 California. EPA. Office of Environmental Health Hazard Assessment. _Chemicals Known to the State to Cause Cancer or Reproductive Toxicity. _February 5,

154 Bisphenol A Exposure: Human Risk and Health Policy; Author links open overlay panelCherylErlerDNP, RNaJulieNovakDNSc, RN, CPNP, FAANPb; Journal of Pediatric Nursing Volume 25, Issue 5, October 2010, Pages 400-407; https://www.sciencedirect.com/science/article/abs/pii/S0882596309001407

155 Bisphenol A, Hypertension, and Cardiovascular Diseases: Epidemiological, Laboratory, and Clinical Trial Evidence. Han C1, Hong YC2,3,4.; Curr Hypertens Rep. 2016 Feb;18(2):11. doi: 10.1007/s11906-015-0617-2.; https://www.ncbi.nlm.nih.gov/pubmed/26781251

156 The Toxic Effects BPA on Fetuses, Infants, and Children; Mujtaba Ellahi and Mamoon ur Rashid; October 11th 2016Reviewed: March 30th 2017Published: June 7th 2017; DOI: 10.5772/intechopen.68896; https://www.intechopen. com/books/bisphenol-a-exposure-and-health-risks/ the-toxic-effects-bpa-on-fetuses-infants-and-children

157 Jensen R. Pornographic lives. Violence Against Women. 1995;1(1):32-54. doi:10.1177/1077801295001001003

158 Thomas Lewis, Fari Amini, and Richard Lannon have written A General Theory of Love (New York: Vintage Books, 2000)

159 Italian men suffer 'sexual anorexia' after Internet porn use, but condition is reversible, experts say; https://www.ansa.it/web/notizie/ rubriche/english/2011/02/24/visualizza_new.html_1583160579.html

160 Excessive Porn Consumption Can Cause Erectile Dysfunction – Myth or Truth? Takeesha Roland-Jenkins, MS | October 6, 2017; http://www.brainblogger.com/2017/10/06/excessive-porn- consumption-can-cause-erectile-dysfunction-myth-or-truth/

161 Your Brain on Drugs: Dopamine and Addiction; David Hirschman; 07 September, 2010; https://bigthink.com/going-mental/ your-brain-on-drugs-dopamine-and-addiction

162 Matthew Christman, M.D., staff urologist, Naval Medical Center, San Diego; Joseph Alukal, M.D., director, male reproductive health, New York University, New York City; May 12, 2017, presentation, American Urological Association annual meeting, Boston

163 Schultz W. Reward signaling by dopamine neurons. Neuroscientist. 2001;7(4):293-302. doi:10.1177/107385840100700406

164 Morrison et al. The Relationship between Excessive Internet Use and Depression: A Questionnaire-Based Study of 1,319 Young People and Adults. Psychopathology, 2010; 43 (2): 121 DOI: 10.1159/000277001

165 Pornography's Influence on Sexual Intimacy; Kevin B Skinner Ph.D.; Inside Porn Addiction; https://www. psychologytoday.com/us/blog/inside-porn-addiction/201201/ pornographys-influence-sexual-intimacy

166 Kate Daine, Keith Hawton, Vinod Singaravelu, Anne Stewart, Sue Simkin, Paul Montgomery. The Power of the Web: A Systematic Review of Studies of the Influence of the Internet on Self-Harm and

Suicide in Young People. PLoS ONE, 2013; 8 (10): e77555 DOI: 10.1371/journal.pone.0077555

167 Winstanley CA, Olausson P, Taylor JR, Jentsch JD. Insight into the relationship between impulsivity and substance abuse from studies using animal models. Alcohol Clin Exp Res. 2010;34(8):1306-1318. doi:10.1111/j.1530-0277.2010. 01215.x

168 M. Liu, L. Wu, S. Yao, Dose-response association of screen time-based sedentary behaviour in children and adolescents and depression: a meta-analysis of observational studies, Br J Sports Med, 50 (20) (2016), pp. 1252-1258

169 Pantic I. Online social networking and mental health. Cyberpsychol Behav Soc Netw. 2014;17(10):652-657. doi:10.1089/cyber.2014.0070

170 K.A. McLaughlin, K. King, Developmental trajectories of anxiety and depression in early adolescence J Abnorm Child Psychol, 43 (2) (2015), pp. 311-323

171 R.C. Kessler, G.P. Amminger, S. Aguilar-Gaxiola, J. Alonso, S. Lee, T. Üstün, Age of onset of mental disorders: a review of recent literature, Curr Opin Psychiatry, 20 (4) (2007), pp. 359-364

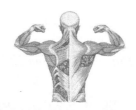

ABOUT THE AUTHOR

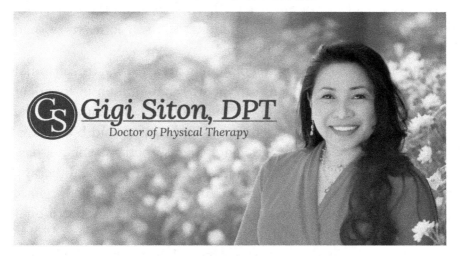

Dr. Gigi Siton, DPT
www.gigisiton.com

Dr. Gigi Siton, DPT, founder, and CEO of Holistic Physical Therapy, has a doctorate in physical therapy with almost thirty years of clinical experience. She is the author of multiple books: (1) *"THE SEXY ART OF HIGH-HEEL WALKING": How To Wear High Heels Pain-free*; (2) *"YOUR BODY IS A SELF-HEALING MACHINE"* Trilogy - *"Your Body Is A Self- Healing Machine"* Trilogy - Book 1: *"Understanding Epigenetics – Why It Is Important To Know";* Book 2: *"Understanding the Anatomy of Epigenetics";* Book 3: *"Understanding How Epigenetics Heals You."* She was one of the speakers at the Personal Improvement Symposium, Harvard University Faculty Club, on

September 20 & 12, 2017. For almost eight years at her Holistic Physical Therapy Clinic, she has taught a monthly class called *"Nutritional Bootcamp: A Practical Class on Epigenetics 101."*

She finished her Doctorate in Physical Therapy from Simmons College, Boston, MA, and a Bachelor of Science in Physical Therapy from De La Salle University, Cavite, Philippines. She also has a Bachelor of Science in Psychology from the University of Santo Tomas, Manila, Philippines. She is also a Nutritional Therapy Practitioner (NTP).

She has worked in inpatient acute care, neuro, stroke, spinal cord injuries, post-surgical orthopedic rehabilitation in inpatient and outpatient settings, labor and delivery, neonatal babies, inpatient and outpatient pediatrics, and wound and burn care, school setting, cardiac rehab acute, and outpatient. For the past seventeen years, she has worked in an outpatient physical therapy setting for acute and chronic pain management, pelvic floor rehab, orthopedic rehab, vertigo rehab, sports medicine, and nutritional medicine.

In 2013, she finally opened her own Holistic Physical Therapy Clinic north of Houston. It is a holistic practice that addresses the root cause of the problem, not just the symptoms. She believes that this holistic physical therapy approach is the cornerstone of any comprehensive and holistic health program. The six keys to holistic health and healing are: nutritional, physical, emotional, social, environmental, and spiritual. When your body works the way that nature intended, your spirit soars—and therefore, so do you.

Her physical therapy style is a combination of Eastern philosophy with Western medicine training and sensibilities. She has further enhanced her skills with years of training in traditional physical therapy interventions combined with additional advanced training in a myofascial trigger point release, acupuncture, internal Qigong, yoga, Pilates on mat and the reformer, whole-body vibration therapy, energy medicine, manual manipulation, visceral manipulation, kinesiotaping, and TRX with sports medicine.

Texas Monthly Magazine named her Five-Star Physical Therapist two years in a row and a recipient of the 2015 Houston Medical Awards for Best Physical Therapy Clinic.

In 1989, she was directly hired to work for Conroe Regional Hospital as a Licensed Physical Therapist in an acute care setting. She came from very humble beginnings. She is the tenth child of twelve children from the southern island of the Philippines called Mindanao. She has eight sisters and three brothers. Oroquieta City is her beloved hometown, where all her passion and inner core started. Her father was a criminal lawyer, state prosecutor, and dean of the College of Law. He was brutally assassinated on August 29, 1985. Her mother was also an educator with a master's in elementary education. She died in her sleep from a broken heart two and a half years after her father's passing. With God's blessing, all her siblings have finished college and post-graduate studies. They all have successful careers.

She is a single mother who loves spending time with her two daughters, Ally and Victoria. She is an eternal student, a voracious reader, loves to dance and travel. She loves meeting people and making them smile and helping them feel better about themselves.

Her mission in life: *"I intend to make people feel better about themselves because they met me."*

CPSIA information can be obtained
at www.ICGtesting.com
Printed in the USA
LVHW050858010721
691592LV00001B/2/J